Trouble Talking

Trouble Talking

*The Realities of Communication,
Language, and Speech Disorders*

Daniel R. Boone

ROWMAN & LITTLEFIELD
Lanham • Boulder • New York • London

Published by Rowman & Littlefield
A wholly owned subsidary of The Rowman & Littlefield Publishing Group, Inc.
4501 Forbes Boulevard, Suite 200, Lanham, Maryland 20706
www.rowman.com

Unit A, Whitacre Mews, 26-34 Stannary Street, London SE11 4AB

British Library Cataloguing in Publication Information Available

Library of Congress Cataloging-in-Publication Data

Names: Boone, Daniel R., author.
Title: Trouble talking : the realities of communication, language, and speech
    disorders / Daniel R. Boone.
Description: Lanham : Rowman & Littlefield, [2018] | Includes bibliographical
    references and index.
Identifiers: LCCN 2017052854 (print) | LCCN 2017054415 (ebook) | ISBN
    9781538110386 (Electronic) | ISBN 9781538110379 (cloth : alk. paper)
Subjects: | MESH: Speech Disorders—therapy | Language Disorders—therapy |
    Speech Therapy | Language Therapy | Case Reports
Classification: LCC RC427 (ebook) | LCC RC427 (print) | NLM WL 340.3 | DDC
    616.85/506—dc23
LC record available at https://lccn.loc.gov/2017052854

♾™ The paper used in this publication meets the minimum requirements of American
National Standard for Information Sciences—Permanence of Paper for Printed Library
Materials, ANSI/NISO Z39.48-1992.

Printed in the United States of America

Contents

~

Introduction

In *Trouble Talking: The Realities of Communication, Language, and Speech Disorders*, I take a fascinating look at many speech pathologies, the people who have them, and their effects on their families and the people around them. Each of the brief stories told here, anecdotal tales, were true clinical or situational events observed directly by me. All names and locations have been changed to protect patient identification.

The ability to speak is one of the most important abilities that separate the human from the animal world.[1] The power of language (both spoken and written) is unique to humanity for punctuating memory, for managing present needs, and for planning future events. In spoken language, the dialogue is between a speaker and a listener who both speak the same language. Likewise, in written language, effective communication requires that both writer and reader use the same language code. However, in communication disorders, the speaker's compromised verbal message has great impact on the appropriateness of the listener's response. As the patient struggles to speak, the listener often does not know how to react. Also, for many head-injury patients who experience a sudden loss of their previous abilities to write and to read, there is a serious compromise in effective communication.

Here you will find a variety of brief encounters between speaker and listener. Some of the particular situations were experienced by the patient while he or she was in speech therapy. Other tales are direct observations of difficulties a person with a communication disorder experienced while reacting in the real world. Some of the tales were told by patients or their families looking back at how their communication struggles affected everything they hoped to do. Similar to stories told by Sacks of experiences of neuropsychiatric patients,[2] this collection of stories brings together dozens of faulty speech episodes that are simultaneously humorous, heartfelt, disturbing, and insightful. For the reader unfamiliar with communication disorders, we will take a brief look at the disorder followed by a glimpse of the person who had difficulty talking in a particular situation. When speakers speak differently from their listeners, some listeners react inappropriately.

The difference in talking, such as someone speaking with a stutter, can shape the response of the listener to, for example, look the other way or say the problematic word. Or the unexpected repetition of a person with aphasia who keeps repeating the same phrase (like a woman in one of my stories who could only say "damn shoes") may force the listener to untangle the utterance for some literal meaning. Or the faulty speech of a man with Parkinson's disease may force his listeners to guess at what he is trying to say. Or patients with dementia, who may look like everyone else their age, may give an unrelated or bizarre response to a stranger's question. Or the woman who has lost her voice cannot make her feelings known on the phone to her son who is somewhere away from home. Almost all of these patient-types are often seen by medically oriented and university-based speech-language pathologists.

Although I have been a speech-language pathologist (SLP) for many decades, I am now but one of a growing number of SLPs practicing in our discipline. In 2017, there were over 191,000 audiologists and speech-language pathologist members of the American Speech-Language-Hearing Association (ASHA). The clinically certified clinicians in ASHA are about equally divided into two work settings: (1) preschool and school programs; or (2) medical/university clinical programs. There are more than 30 million Americans with speech-language-voice disorders related to various causes: hearing loss, developmental delay, neurological disorders, brain injury, intellectual disabilities, drug abuse, physical impairments such as cleft lip or palate, or vocal abuse or misuse. Most of these various causes of communication disorders are treatable by speech-language pathologists (SLPs) and specialists from other professional disciplines. After identifying causation and planning treatment of the disorder, the usual goal of speech therapy is to improve the communication between speaker and listener.

Again for the reader, the focus of many of the stories is the impact of the patient's talking problem on his or her listeners, who usually expect the speaker to understand and speak the same way they do. When speakers speak differently, they sometimes are negatively shaping the listener's response.

And, of course, negative listener response may often negatively shape the future behavior of the patient.

Unique to the stories in *Trouble Talking* is the range of ages of children and adults who collectively represent a diversity of communication disorders. This diversity of patient type in the stories is directly related to my working as a medically oriented speech-language pathologist in a series of different clinical settings (including private practice). My first clinical experience in speech pathology was helping young men with aphasia, who had experienced devastating head wounds during the Korean War, learn to talk again. Then, in graduate school and beyond, I was fortunate to work for seven years in a chronic-disease hospital in Cleveland, where I treated people with stroke-induced aphasia and other patients with degenerative diseases (like multiple sclerosis or Parkinson's disease), who struggled with their motor-speech disorders. Later I saw patients in a children's rehabilitation center, university speech and hearing clinics, and a university hospital communication disorders clinic.

These diverse tales are organized into five different kinds of communication disorders, each with its own chapter: chapter 1, Tales of Aphasia; chapter 2, Tales of Dementia; chapter 3, Tales of Neurogenic Disorders; chapter 4, Tales of Voice Disorders; chapter 5, Tales of Speech Pathology. After the presentation of the stories in each particular chapter, we consider questions that the stories have generated. In the final chapter, chapter 6, Management of Communication Disorders, we offer some useful summary discussion of both short-term and long-term strategies for improving patient communication.

The brief tales of our patients with communication disorders can be found in these chapters:

Chapter 1: Tales of Aphasia. These are true stories about adult patients who acquired some kind of brain damage from either head trauma or stroke. The language problems of aphasia may show in difficulties understanding spoken language or in reading, with obvious difficulties in speaking or writing.

Chapter 2: Tales of Dementia. Patients with dementia, usually of the Alzheimer's type, are described in various living situations. These patients often give an unrelated or bizarre response to questions. Of particular interest in this chapter are the coping strategies used in the early days of an emerging dementia by both the patient and family.

Chapter 3: Tales of Neurogenic Disorders. Faulty communication situations are described in this chapter for a wide variety of neurologically impaired patients (cerebral palsy, Parkinson's disease, head injury, etc.) For example, a middle-aged man with Lou Gehrig's disease (ALS) describes his struggle to speak and to swallow.

Chapter 4: Tales of Voice Disorders. These stories about a few voice patients were selected from a large clinical file of children and adults with voice disorders. For example, a middle-aged woman complained after the removal of her larynx (laryngectomy) that the thing she missed the most without a voice was her ability to cry or to laugh.

Chapter 5: Tales of Speech Pathology. The first three stories in this chapter illustrate coping with stuttering by a young child, a professor, and a sea captain. We then appreciate the transition of a male-to-female transgender woman as she feminizes her communication style. A young man is described with elective mutism in a state prison, followed by a final tale of faulty communication between a handicapped pilot flying his Cessna with the surprise help of this author.

Chapter 6: Management of Communication Disorders. In this summary chapter, we look at things family members and other listeners can do to improve a patient's communication effectiveness. An initial strategy would be to look for a speech-language pathologist (SLP), particularly one with extensive clinical experience in the specific area of the patient's problem. Then there is a need for planning long-term patient management by requesting input from audiologists, speech-language pathologists, special education teachers, otolaryngologists, neurologists, and other rehabilitation specialists.

When you've completed reading *Trouble Talking*, I hope you'll agree that this isn't a book about disorders, but about a group of courageous individuals doing their best to communicate with one another. I hope their stories, or "tales," as I call them here, inspire you and give you a deeper understanding of the power of language—and an appreciation of the human heart.

~

CHAPTER ONE

Tales of Aphasia

As was discussed in the "Introduction," a distinct feature of human beings is the use of language, particularly the ability to talk and understand the speech of others. Together with our human spoken language skill is written language, the ability to read and to write. Aphasia is characterized as the partial or complete loss of both spoken and written language abilities, usually the result of an injury to the brain from either head trauma or a vascular stroke. A great portion of my career has been spent as a speech-language pathologist (SLP) working with adult patients with aphasia.

The type of aphasia the patient has is related to the site and extent of insult to the brain. In general, aphasia develops from lesions to the left cerebral hemisphere (left brain). Brain lesions that are more forwardly positioned produce what is known as a non-fluent aphasia, or expressive aphasia, characterized by extreme complications in saying words, while retaining fairly good understanding of what others are saying. More posterior brain lesions often produce fluent aphasia, or receptive aphasia, in which the patient may speak with a jumbled or jargony speech, often completely unaware of his or her jargon and also showing some difficulty understanding the speech of others. Most people with aphasia actually end up performing somewhere in between the extremes of non-fluent and fluent aphasia, with their problem often labeled as receptive-expressive aphasia.

While the extent and type of aphasia is determined by the site of the brain lesion, how well the patient communicates is usually determined by his or her personality and by the reactions of the people surrounding the patient.

Most people speak to express their ideas, their needs, their feelings; patients with aphasia, even with their compromised speech, speak for the same reasons. My attempt in this chapter is to lead the reader to appreciate the differences and communication struggles of the adult person with aphasia. As I recount some speaking situations and conditions, they may appear humorous and produce laughter. We are not laughing at the patient, but rather at the reactions of the listener who takes literally the patient's verbal responses in particular situations. On the other hand, the reader may experience an emotional tear while reading about someone struggling in their recovery from aphasia. Although most of the following aphasia tales occurred dating back to the 1950s, all names and locales have been changed to protect patient identity.

I begin with the aphasia tale "The Thank You," a story that had a great impact on me as a clinician over a lifetime career as a speech-language pathologist. I then tell the story "Damn Shoes," a fun example of a non-fluent aphasic woman cheering at a football game. Like many people with non-fluent aphasia, her perseverative responses of the same few words were taken literally by those surrounding her in the stadium. Two other talking tales, "Away" and "Water, Water, Water," provide an amusing perspective on how the typical listener responds to the repetitions of non-fluent aphasia patients. A retired airline pilot with fluent aphasia describes in his own jargon speech, the problems he once had landing a DC-10 in "Circling Over Dallas." In "Your Penchant for Apples?" the reader will experience some of the frustrations shared by a patient and the clinician who was attempting to evaluate the patient's newly acquired aphasia. From the many aphasia group therapy sessions that I have facilitated, I selected one narrative in particular, "Honolulu Annie," which illustrates some fun interaction in aphasia group therapy. In "Looking Back at Our People with Aphasia," we take a review look at each tale and how it might answer some questions about aphasia.

⌒

Tale 1: The Thank You

During the Korean War, I worked as a language retraining instructor in the aphasia clinic at the Long Beach VA Hospital in California. The majority of our speech-language patients at that time were young men who had sustained some kind of head injury on the battlefield. One such patient, whom I will always remember, was Louie, a 19-year-old Mexican American who fell in combat while carrying a large Browning automatic rifle. When he fell, he dropped the gun, discharging a bullet through his left eye, destroying much of his left forehead, skull, and the anterior brain behind it. His injury produced a right-sided paralysis (hemiplegia) and a profound non-fluent aphasia. For six months before transferring to our VA hospital, he had been in a service hospital in Japan, unable to utter a single word. When I first saw him, his aphasia was about seven months old.

I went to visit him on the aphasia ward for the first time. His chart noted that he had good comprehension of both English and Spanish, but was unable to speak or write. My quick testing of his ability to read and understand what was spoken revealed good function, confirming the chart notation (which often with aphasia assumes falsely that the patient has no problem in understanding). Louie demonstrated a severe expressive aphasia. When asked to say a simple word like "ball," he could only awkwardly purse his lips and make no sound. He could not successfully follow any of my attempts at modeling, to show him how to say a simple word.

On my second visit with Louie, however, he was able to imitate a word. We had practiced humming, which he could do now with some ease. We then looked in a mirror, and I demonstrated for Louie that if we were humming and slowly opened our mouth, a word like "ma" would come out. He was able to do it, and he celebrated his success by repeating the word "ma" again and again. Other patients on the ward and his mother (who visited every day) cheerfully joined in our therapy program, encouraging him to continually flaunt his new accomplishment.

Once we had the beginning /m/ sound, I introduced Louie to a spiral-bound notebook. On the top of the first page, we wrote in big capital letters the /m/ sound and underneath it, the word "ma." Within a day or so, we had a list of 15 words, all beginning with the /m/ sound that Louie was able to say without much prompting: "ma, mom, morn, man, more, main, me, mean, many, mama, moon, my, may, make, meat." At the bottom of the page were /m/ phrases like "many men on the moon."

Once one sound had been mastered and Louie could say it on request with very little struggle, we would move on to another sound, such as /p/. Each page in the notebook had the practice words at the top and phrases and then sentences below them. We were soon able to introduce short phrases and sentences without using our practice notebook lists of single words. Toward the end of six months, Louie was able to read aloud some captions and headlines from a daily newspaper.

When I left the Long Beach VA for graduate school in Ohio, I did not see Louie again until eleven years later. He appeared at a national convention on a panel of "recovered aphasic patients." I sat in the audience listening to each one of the people who had recovered from aphasia. I marveled with great pride as Louie, in near normal speech, told his recovery story. At the session break, I got up from my seat and walked toward the speaker's platform. Louie saw me and walked down to greet me (he walked with a cane because of his continued right-sided paralysis). As we met in the aisle, I could see our old spiral-bound notebook in his left hand (he had shown it to the audience). For a moment, neither of us said anything. Instead, we embraced one another like the long-lost friends that we were. Finally, he looked at me and said through his tears, "I just want to thank you for helping me learn to talk again." No "thank you" ever meant so much to me as that one.

Many patients with aphasia can make functional recoveries if they have enough speech-language therapy. The VA in the early 1950s was able to offer Louie an exceptional amount of needed therapy. He received three hours of group and individual speech-language therapy daily for almost two years. Besides his speech and language retraining, he had physical and vocational therapy. His excellent motivation helped him to make the most of his therapeutic opportunities. Despite his right-side paralysis (hemiplegia), loss of one eye, and slight residuals of expressive aphasia, he built a wonderful life for himself; he married, had three children, and was employed for many years by McDonnell Douglas, building commercial airliners until he retired. For many years, I looked forward to receiving his annual Christmas card with those same meaningful words, "Thank you."

～

Tale 2: Damn Shoes

The "star" of this narrative is a 44-year-old woman, a WAC veteran of World War II, who was a non-fluent aphasia patient in the Long Beach VA aphasia clinic. She was diagnosed as having "Broca's aphasia" (her predominant problem was the inability to speak). She became well known in the neurology section of the hospital for her inability to say anything but the perseverative simple phrase "damn shoes." She would repeat the nonsensical phrase with differential inflections. For example, if asked if she wanted a home-pass for the coming weekend, she would reply with an enthusiastic "damn shoes," complete with all the happy-voice inflection that would confirm her desire to go home for a few days. If I asked, "Do you like the coffee on the ward?" her negative-voice inflection would say "no" as she repeated "damn shoes."

We will call her Mary Lou. She appeared to have no arm or leg weakness, her only apparent deficit being the severe expressive aphasia that limited her to say only "damn shoes" with perfectly normal-sounding inflections.

One of the more pleasant tasks I had as a young speech-language pathologist at one veteran's hospital in the early 1950s was to accompany our aphasic patients to various recreational programs. The internal programs included meeting with a visiting movie star every other week (Loretta Young, Doris Day, and Kathryn Grayson, among others). Recreational programs outside the hospital grounds included deep-sea fishing, picnics, and various professional athletic events. Another speech clinician and I would accompany about twenty-five patients, most of whom had some form of aphasia, on a bus to an arena, stadium, or other event destination.

Mary Lou frequented these field trips. One Sunday afternoon, we visited the Los Angeles Coliseum with tickets for row 35 near the 40-yard line to see the Los Angeles Rams against the Chicago Bears. The game was billed as "A battle between Bob Waterfield of the Rams and Sid Luckman of the Bears." Mary Lou was a real Rams fan, and stood up and hollered loudly for every Ram advance and opportunity. The problem was that all she hollered was "damn shoes!" Throughout the first quarter, I watched as the people seated in the rows ahead continually looked back to see who kept yelling "damn shoes" on nearly every play. Finally, the man seated directly in front of us could stand it no longer. He stood up, turned around, and exclaimed, "Listen, lady, so Sid Luckman's a Jew!" Then he added, "Can he help it if he's the best player out there?"

The aphasic patient who perseverates on the same few words will often encounter a surprise response from his or her listeners, who are reacting literally to what is continually being said. In this case, the "damn shoes" had no literal meaning, so the listener took it upon himself to assume that Mary Lou was berating the ethnicity of a rival team's star player. These kinds of word perseverations are more commonly used by patients with an expressive aphasia rather than by patients with other types of aphasia.

⌒

Tale 3: Away

Similar to Mary Lou, who could only say "damn shoes," Otto with his severe aphasia could only say, "away, away, away." He would repeat the word with various meaningful inflections. If he was happy, it could be heard in the sound of his voice. If he was angry, his mood showed itself with an angry "away." He presented a great challenge to the professional staff and to his family and friends, all of whom often took his "away" literally. The early management of Otto's recovery from aphasia was thwarted by the misinterpretation by others, who thought that Otto was never happy wherever he happened to be.

As a retired insurance man, Otto was used to making decisions and influencing others to follow his recommendations. So when the paramedics came to his home in the early morning hours following his stroke, his remark, "away, away," was reasonable due to the urgent necessity to leave his lakefront home for the hospital. Once admitted to his hospital room, his wife arrived, only to be greeted with "away." She likely either answered him with some description of his illness and the need for a probable long hospital stay, or interpreted his "away" as a bluntly uttered dismissal, in which case she may have responded accordingly.

During Otto's days in the hospital, ward personnel and occasional visitors were always greeted with "away, away, away." Most everyone countered with something like, "Don't worry, you'll be going home soon." At his discharge planning conference, his wife alleged, "If you'd just listen to the man, you could tell that he won't be happy until he goes home." Otto's rehabilitation was consequently planned for outpatient physical therapy aimed at working on his paralyzed right arm and leg, and speech-language pathology services to focus on his aphasia.

On the day of his hospital discharge, his wife drove their car to the front door of the hospital. Otto, in a wheelchair pushed by a nurse, was happily repeating "away!" As he got in the car, his "aways" became louder and even sounded happier. As soon as they arrived home, his wife wheeled him out to the front veranda overlooking the lake. Otto looked out, gesturing with a sweeping motion of his normal left arm, and in a crying voice said, "away, away." According to his wife, who witnessed the scene, Otto's daughter answered him with a cry, "But, Daddy, you're home now, there's no other place to go."

As Otto experienced some recovery from aphasia, he eventually reduced his "away" repetitions. His leg function improved a bit, allowing him to ambulate easily with a cane. His right arm and hand remained partially paralyzed, but he was successfully trained to write with his normal left hand. He received six months of successful speech-language therapy. Otto and his wife joined a university aphasia support group, where they enjoyed sharing with others the many unfortunate reactions they experienced when all he could say was "away." Today, Otto enjoys fully functional, relatively normal speech. "Away" has disappeared.

~

Tale 4: Water, Water, Water

Similar to the woman who could only say "damn shoes" and Otto with his one-word "away," Helen could only say "water." Helen, an associate dean at the University Hospital College of Nursing, loves to tell students of the frustrating time she had following a stroke that sent her to the hospital, only able to say one word, "water." She enjoys laughing about it now, but at the time of her hospital stay, it brought her nothing but misery.

Helen was the best known patient on the rehabilitation ward at University Hospital, because prior to her stroke she had been the associate dean of the College of Nursing. Many of the ward nurses and aides knew her from previous courses they had taken with her. Helen was a close friend to many. There was nothing any shift of nurses wouldn't do for Helen. Her every wish was their command.

Helen's expressive aphasia left her with very good comprehension of what others said, but with a total inability to respond with any word other than "water." "Water" was her response each time anyone greeted her, and through appropriate inflection, she could convey her moods.

When each new shift of nurses came on duty and visited patients, priority was given to Helen. She would greet them with a friendly "water, water, water." The nursing staff, along with others who came to visit her, would assume she was thirsty, refill her water pitcher, and offer her a glass. Rather than drinking the water, Helen would respond with a perturbed-sounding "water!"

Fortunately for Helen, in a few weeks she experienced a near spontaneous recovery from aphasia. When she had recovered to a point where she could comfortably recount her time spent hospitalized, she recalled one night on the ward: Desperate for the nurse to bring her a much needed bedpan, Helen's compromised speech abilities got her no relief for her distended bladder. "Water, water," she would say and in came the nurse with the "cause" of her predicament, another pitcher of water.

• It is of interest to note that the perseverate word in this story and the word repetitions in the two previous tales were all said with varying inflections. In aphasia, the inflectional rhythm of perseverations is still there in the sound of the voice, reflecting the mood of the patient, such as anger, questioning, happiness, concern, and other mood states.

⌒

Tale 5: Circling Over Dallas

Captain Dan had been a commercial airline pilot from the time he was 28 years old until he was forced to retire at age 60. About five years after leaving the airline, Captain Dan had a stroke that left him with a profound fluent aphasia. When first seen in our aphasia clinic, the captain appeared as a handsome older man, free of any motor weakness of arm or leg, but he spoke with a rather profound jargon. Typical of this kind of jargon aphasia patient, he was unaware of his own speech errors. Consequently, he spoke freely with normal speech rhythm, but his language contained many neologisms (made-up words) spoken in a twisted word order. There were, however, enough occasional real words that a listener could grossly understand what he was talking about. Captain Dan had difficulty following spoken commands, and his reading ability was dramatically reduced from what had obviously been a superior level in his work as an airline pilot. The brief interview that follows was recorded about five months after the onset of his stroke.

Boone: "They tell me, Captain, that you were an airline pilot."
Captain D: "Well, here's a granching thought that I flew the big one, starting with DC 4s and throttling the props cathings for a living. Stayed with the pilot casing all the way through the sixes and sedners to the DC-10, which by the way, was the finest coredevil that evet too mover the country and promorthing the world. She could let the conlens if any crube to confusart the landing."
Boone: "You were a captain flying DC-10s? I've enjoyed flying as a passenger in them."
Captain D: "Yes, well the proudest outfit of the Douglas parade was the ten that could go anywhere, but she never made a noise about it. I had one toubler with a tenner when she was about out of fuel circling over Dallas. We had chagened all the trando from New York Kennedy and radio shooting and by the time we go to Dallas, she was weydown with one hell of a staroom over never again. We had no idea that the scarshun tenfa was even torping

to anyone. We couldn't get the bid won when we tried fuging to circling and she selaid you cannot get her down, so we circled over Dallas till our three hungry acalameters were going to run out of kerosenedine."

Boone: "Well, did you ever get to land there?"

Captain D: "Hell, they had a diversification that would put pimples on your belly bashen for the asking for some damn perplastion to set the tenner down on their gladden fallen runway. So I confeerted with the Dallas tow-took her and everybody in het up to Austin."

Captain Dan liked to talk about particular flying events from his career. If he understood the gist of a question, he would often ramble on, looking closely at his listeners' faces to see if they were still interested in what he was saying. He received four months of individual speech-language therapy with heavy emphasis on auditory feedback. In our therapy sessions, we forced him to track closely what was said to him, and we encouraged close self-monitoring of what he said in reply. After discharge from our therapy program, he fortunately found a couple of helpful auditory feedback apps on his laptop computer that required him to listen closely to what he had just said and then repeat it back on his recorder. His self-practice listening efforts proved helpful. I last saw Captain Dan several years ago, and he was speaking with near normal speech, enjoying fishing in his retirement.

∼

Tale 6: Your Penchant for Apples?

The first encounter with a new patient, particularly one with aphasia, is most important for developing a good working relationship between the patient and clinician. Adult patients with aphasia have had a lifetime of using normal language until their precipitating event, such as an accident or stroke. It is important, then, that when they show difficulty speaking, to still approach them with the assumption that they can speak, and that they understand all that is said to them. I learned over time to approach new aphasic patients, who had been referred to me by their doctors, with this kind of approach: "Good morning. I am Doctor Boone. I work here in the hospital with patients who may be having trouble talking. I wanted to check with you. Are you having any trouble speaking or understanding what is said to you?" A patient who has no problem will not be offended by such a question. The patient with aphasia will demonstrate his problem when attempting to answer the question.

In my early days as a graduate assistant seeing patients with aphasia for the first time in hospitals, I remember a few awkward situations like this "apples" story. I had been requested to see Walter, a 64-year-old business executive, in his private room for his problems with receptive-expressive aphasia. When making our first visit for such an evaluation, we usually brought along a small testing kit that included pictures, a few objects, and paper and pencil. Usually after the first visit, we would schedule the patient for a full standardized examination for aphasia. When I visited Walter, the first thing I wanted to find out was his ability to repeat words after me, which would give some direction as to what kind of aphasia he had, as well as give me some idea of what to test first.

As I entered his room carrying my testing kit, he was sitting up in bed looking as if he were reading the morning paper. Many patients with aphasia may look as if they are reading, but may not understand the words they see. In any case, I interrupted him and said, "Good morning, I'm Mister Boone. Your doctor wanted me to see you about your speech. I understand you've been having some trouble talking since your stroke."

Walter put his paper down, took off his reading glasses, and gave me a long look. "I had a few days there where it was hard to talk." He looked at me again for a long time before asking, "What is it you want to know?"

"Well, it looks like your words are coming out pretty well." Attempting to take control of the situation, but making no attempt to get to know him as a person, I said, "Let's just see how you can say things after me." As he kept staring intently at me, I became a bit flustered and quickly added, "You say after me what I say. Are you ready?" Hardly waiting for his reply, I said in a loud voice the first word to repeat: "Apple."

The man threw his newspaper down on the bed and asked, "What's going on here?"

Flustered by his obvious annoyance but hanging in with the examination, I continued, "Can you say 'apple'? Let me hear you say 'apple.'"

"What the hell is this penchant you have for apples?" Walter stared me down, waiting for my response.

I replied, not thinking, "I don't have anything for apples, sir, I just wanted to find out if you could say it."

"Well, son, there are all kinds of apples: There are Winesap and Delicious and Granny Smith. What is going on in your mind about apples?"

My examination attempt was a failure, and we just talked for a few moments. He dominated me as the gray-haired executive, not tolerating well the intrusion into his room by the young male student therapist.

The important lesson I learned from my apple encounter with Walter (who probably had experienced a spontaneous recovery from aphasia *before* I saw him) is always to preface your speech examinations by getting to know the patient as a person rather than as someone with a clinical condition. Another thing I learned from this encounter that I always remembered throughout my teaching years: always have patience with young people who are learning a clinical craft, and demonstrate tolerance for their mistakes.

～

Tale 7: Honolulu Annie

Most speech-language therapy for adults who have acquired aphasia is provided on an individual basis between the patient and the speech-language pathologist (SLP). If a sufficient number of aphasic patients are available, group therapy should also be scheduled. The clinician may incorporate within the group therapy session a family member, a speech aide, or a student SLP. Therapy emphasis is given to encouraging the patient to communicate, using words, gestures, pictures, objects, or anything that will "get the message across." Increasing communication effectiveness, even without saying words per se (perhaps by facial expression or gesture), is the aphasia therapy goal. My own particular therapy bias was heavy on listening and talking, with little emphasis given to reading and writing tasks.

From my early days at the Long Beach VA Hospital, I always supplemented individual therapy with group therapy. We would typically limit the size of the group from four to seven aphasia patients, with the group coordinated by myself and an assistant (usually a graduate student). We kept as little structure to our groups as possible, encouraging spontaneous communication, often punctuated with patient laughter. The group therapy leader had to be sure that all patients communicated at their top ability level within the session. This talking tale, "Honolulu Annie," describes briefly the communication thrusts of six aphasia group patients reacting to Annie and her fun hula dance while sitting in a wheelchair.

We had six adult folks in the group that day: Annie, age 71, a retired Hawaiian show woman; Bill, 75, a pilot friend of Clark Gable who had lived in Tucson; Joe, 52, a mathematics college professor who could say nothing but "pretty good"; Keith, 77, a big band piano player who had played in the Harry James orchestra; Priscilla, 63, who had managed a coffee shop; and Marie, 81, a housewife who lived for her home flower garden. They were a mixture of people not only with different backgrounds but also with two kinds of aphasia (expressive aphasia and receptive-expressive aphasia). This excerpt of a fun group session was video-recorded on the day Annie had promised to come to the group session wearing her Hawaiian grass skirt complete with floral lei.

Boone: "Look at Annie sitting there like Hilo Hattie." Boone points to Annie wearing her grass skirt and sitting in her wheelchair.

Bill: "God damn and looks like Hilo Hattie to me."

Joe: "Pretty good, pretty good" (smiling big and gesturing with his normal left arm and hand).

Boone: "Hilo Hattie? How many remember her?" Several patients did remember the performer Hilo Hattie.

Marie: She begins to tell Annie, "Well, you should be, as I remember, your flowers are gorgeous and . . ." (searching for words). Two student clinicians wheel in a spinet piano.

Many of us are all talking at once, but Keith says in a louder voice, "Music, music. I hear a song coming on." He gets out of his chair and walks with a slight limp to the piano. He strums the piano keys and drums out what sounds like the "Hawaiian War Chant," with a fast pulsating beat. Joe and Bill mix their "God damn, it's going to be" and "pretty good" with a lot of laughter. Priscilla looks a bit confused as to what is going on, but begins tapping her left foot to Keith's piano rhythms.

Boone: "Priscilla, what can we have to drink at a Hawaiian party?" She has difficulty answering. Priscilla has right hemiplegia, but like Annie lifts her left arm high and makes circular movements with her fingers.

Annie: "Oh, boy," and she begins singing "lawanna, lawanna, kanna" and picks up the beat with Keith repeating the same Hawaiian-sounding words. The whole group spontaneously reacts to Keith's playing and Annie's singing with other group members saying, "Pretty good," "I don't know," "God damn, it's Hilo Hattie," "Oh, darn I love this so."

Marie: "Annie, can you dance with your singing?"

Boone encourages the group to look at Annie as she begins the best hula dance in a wheelchair that anyone has ever seen. She thrusts out her left leg in a seductive circle, tries to sway her hips to the piano music, and goes through all the hand motions needed with her good left hand.

Annie: Doing the hula the best she can, sings, "lawanna, lawanna, kanna . . ."

A critical observer might view this session and ask, "That is group therapy?" I would have to answer that it was a marvelous session, one that allowed each patient to participate in a spontaneous musical event. We had the piano music, the wheelchair song and dance, and the people clapping and laughing in response to Annie's hula. That morning, the six of them were people, not patients.

⌒

Looking Back at Our People with Aphasia

I have told many of these tales over the years to students in classes and workshops. Many of these students were unfamiliar with the problem of aphasia, and the feedback I received was that the tales piqued their desire to know more about aphasia. I received similar responses from several dozen lay readers whom I had asked to review the unpublished manuscript for readability and for any feedback suggestions they might have. The most prevalent feedback item was, again, that after reading the tales, they wanted to know more about aphasia.

In turn, I thought we could learn something more about aphasia by revisiting the tales of the six patients in our individual sessions and the six people in our aphasia group. From our collective feedback, these questions seemed like good ones for starting to appreciate more about aphasia:

- **Do aphasia patients experience two kinds of recovery: spontaneous and from speech therapy?**
- **Do perseverative words like "damn shoes" eventually become less frequent or fade away?**
- **How should listeners respond to the faulty speech responses of people with aphasia?**
- **Does the jargon speech of receptive aphasics retain the accent and melody of normal speech?**
- **Is fostering humanism a primary goal in aphasia group therapy?**

We will let our patient tales guide us in our answers to these frequent questions about aphasia.

Before we look at answers to the questions, we need first to review the three types of aphasia experienced by our 12 patients: There were five people who experienced non-fluent expressive aphasia, five who struggled to find their words with receptive-expressive aphasia, and two men who had some jargon speech related to receptive aphasia. While we can generalize the answers to the questions by considering patient history and by our observations, in chapter 6 we will guide the reader to some literature references that may further support our answers to the questions.

Five Questions about Aphasia

Do aphasia patients experience two kinds of recovery: spontaneous and from speech therapy?

Some patients show a remarkable recovery of receptive and expressive language functions within days or a few weeks after onset, and before receiving any speech therapy. This return of function is known as *spontaneous recovery*.

Helen, the professor of nursing, experienced a recovery of impaired speaking ability before speech therapy could be started. Walter, the insurance man, experienced recovery within three days of his hospital admission. Of some relevance here, both of these patients received needed medical care to reduce the symptoms of their strokes within two hours after the onset of their strokes. Early medical intervention after a stroke can have a direct impact on minimizing symptoms. Keith, the piano player in our aphasia group, was seen initially by us one month after the onset of his stroke; we saw only mild remnants of his receptive aphasia (which had been "severe," according to his letter of referral). All three of these patients are excellent examples of people who experienced spontaneous recovery of compromised language function within a few days or weeks after a stroke.

Three of the people in our aphasia tales did not experience spontaneous recovery. Louie was the most dramatic example of the lack of such a recovery. He had remained in a US Army hospital in Japan for six months, unable to say a single word. After his medical discharge from the army, he was referred to our aphasia clinic at the Long Beach VA Hospital. His remarkable recovery, described in our first aphasia tale, "The Thank You," was the result of intensive speech-language therapy. Mary Lou had experienced a stroke a year before she came to our VA aphasia clinic. Post-stroke, she could only say "damn shoes." Apparently, there was no spontaneous recovery of her ability to speak. Although she improved in socialization with other patients, she was discharged from our program still only able to speak her two nonsense words. After moving to Tucson from Arkansas, Joe, from our aphasia group, came into our university clinic about 18 months after receiving a devastating head injury from an automobile accident. Despite our best efforts in individual therapy, all he could say were the perseverative words, "pretty good." In group therapy, despite his limited speech, he was an active and cooperative participant in all group activities.

The question about two kinds of recovery (spontaneous or from speech therapy), however, is an invalid one. The two types of recovery do not exist independent of one another. For most of our patients, speech therapy was initiated "on top" of any spontaneous improvement. Six other patients in our tales, not mentioned in the above spontaneous recovery discussion, received both individual and group therapy for their receptive-expressive aphasias. Our two men with receptive aphasia each began individual therapy about 30 days after their strokes. Hopefully, their therapies began early enough after onset as possible to take advantage of any possible assistance from spontaneous recovery.

Do perseverative words like "damn shoes" eventually become less frequent or fade away?

Patients with severe expressive aphasia are more likely to be the patients who perseverate saying the same word or phrase. Both Mary Lou with her "damn shoes" and Joe with his "pretty good" came into our therapy program a year or more after the onset of their aphasia. It takes early therapy intervention to eliminate or diminish the occurrence of perseverative words. Neither Mary Lou nor Joe received early therapy. Otto, with his continuous "away" for everything he wanted to say, began speech-language therapy in the hospital within seven days after his stroke. Because his "away" utterances were interpreted by hospital staff to mean that Otto was unhappy with his hospitalization, he was prematurely sent home. However, he continued speech therapy as an outpatient as soon as arrangements could be made. Early efforts using musical patterns of speech with his SLP were successful in eliminating his perseverative "away."

Because of a complete expressive aphasia after the onset of Helen's stroke, she could say nothing other than "water" for a few days. Her "water" response quickly disappeared as she experienced a complete spontaneous recovery within ten days after onset. However, in a follow-up interview a few months later, she reported that during a few stressful situations, she caught herself almost saying "water" again.

The other patients in our aphasia tales did not develop perseverative words. If they were identified during the speech evaluation and first therapy visits, a search was made for some other words the patient could still say. Early therapy efforts focused on intensive practice of the repetition of things the patient could still say beyond the perseveration.

Computer apps (many available and always changing) are helpful, requiring the patient to fill in the blank by saying the missing word that completes an automatic verbal utterance, such as 1-2-3-4-5-6-7-8-9-___; Sunday-Monday-Tuesday-Wednesday-___; it's either hot or ___; north or ___; up and ___; and other automatic word contrasts.

Or the missing word of a well-known song may aid the patient in saying a new word. The SLP sings: "Home, home on the ___"; or "Take me out to the ___"; or "Let me call you ___."

Whenever a blank word is said, it is repeated many times without the initial automatic phrasing before it. Using some kind of automatic word production is an important part of aphasia therapy, and is usually successful in eradicating annoying perseverative words. Effective therapy usually begins with what normal speech the patient can still say, followed by extensive practice using this normal speech.

How should listeners respond to the broken speech responses of people with aphasia?

The reactions of listeners to how and what aphasics are able to say are many and varied. Normal two-way communication is possible because both speaker and listener use the same language. If one of the speakers has aphasia, this two-way model breaks down. The normal speaker, like most people, has been conditioned by a lifetime of both speaker and listener using the same common language. This two-way language can be seriously compromised by aphasia.

Inappropriate listener reactions are most severe for patients with expressive aphasia, as experienced by four patients in our tales (Louie, Bill, Mary Lou, and Helen). An almost unanimous reaction to their lack of appropriate verbal response was the listener talking back in a louder voice with exaggerated slower speech. Louie, with his severe expressive aphasia, was unable to speak for over six months. Looking back at those speechless days, Louie said in a recording, "They all thought I was too dumb to talk. So they would yell at me or tell me to look at their face as they talked. Everybody thought I was deaf." In the aphasia group, Bill, who had in the beginning a severe expressive aphasia, talked about people talking louder to him when he had no speech to answer them. Mary Lou nodded her head in agreement, saying her usual "damn shoes" in a voice that sounded like she agreed. Helen's "water" words were interpreted by most of her hospital visitors as requests for more water. Looking back, Helen found the water experience one of the most difficult things she had to deal with in her recovery from aphasia.

Most of our patients with receptive-expressive aphasia (Otto, Annie, Priscilla, Marie, and Walter) complained of other people speaking too loudly to them. Priscilla and Otto both complained about some people slowing down their rate of speech, which seemed to make it even harder to understand them. Otto described a nurse who always talked to him in baby talk. Annie joined almost everyone in the group in complaining how the people around her were always guessing what she wanted to say. The inability to retrieve

and say words (anomia) is a common problem for receptive-expressive aphasics; it is made worse by the listener guessing and saying the missing word for
the patient. Upon his discharge from the hospital, Walter wrote this note,
which represents a common feeling among people with a disability like aphasia: "The thing that bothered me the most when I had difficulty talking was
hearing some staff refer to me as 'the guy with aphasia in room 223.' Inside,
I was an anxious person wondering if I would ever talk again."

The predominantly receptive aphasic patient is the most challenging for
others to understand. Although these patients have the same kind of peripheral hearing they have always had, they may appear hard of hearing because of
their difficulty understanding the spoken word. Both Captain Dan and Keith
experienced severe receptive aphasia shortly after their strokes. They had difficulty following and understanding what others said. They later reported that
because another person's words had sounded jumbled to them, they closely
watched the speaker's facial expression and tone of voice in a search for meaning. In the beginning, they were unaware of their own jargon speech.

As patients with receptive aphasia begin to recover, their listening confusion begins to lessen. Sentences become less jumbled. The listener is able to
communicate with the patient with far more accuracy and relevance. After
his recovery and listening to prior recordings of his jargon speech, Captain
Dan had this to say: "It sure as hell sounded like my voice doing the talking.
It makes me feel sorry though for the folks who were trying to figure what I
was talking about."

Does the jargon speech of receptive aphasics retain the accent and melody of normal speech?

Before we discuss the question, let's take a brief look at "accent and
melody" of speech. The accent and rhythm flow of a language is known as
prosody. Prosody is deeply rooted in the development of spoken language in
everyone. In the first few months of life, babies around the world basically
sound alike as they make various babble sounds. At five to six months, these
sounds become more differentiated, sounding more like what the baby has
been hearing around him. At nine to ten months, infant jargon begins to
sound like the same prosody of the parent language. The prosody of that
particular language (such as French, Mandarin Chinese, Spanish, etc.) is well
established even before the emergence of the first words. Prosody not only
carries for a lifetime its linguistic message, but the sound of the voice also carries feelings of emotion: happiness, fear, anger, love, uncertainty, and others.

The prosody, or rhythm, of the language is preserved in receptive-expressive
and predominantly receptive aphasia, but not in expressive aphasia. Since

most aphasias are the result of left-brain lesions, apparently the expression of normal prosody is dependent on frontal areas of the left brain. Disturbance to the left frontal brain is the causative site of expressive aphasia (or non-fluent aphasia), and prosody is usually seriously impaired. In both receptive-expressive and predominantly receptive aphasia, the primary language problem is word retrieval and phrase/sentence formulation. What is said is spoken with normal language prosody.

Although Louie made a remarkable recovery from aphasia, his connected speech often lacked a little normal fluency. Bill and Joe had slight changes of melody in their speech. All of our other patients had normal prosody for the words they were able to say. The fluent jargon of Captain Dan is a classic example of jargon words said with meaning and appropriate emotion, all possible by still having normal prosody. Patients with jargon speech in receptive aphasia retain normal speech prosody.

Is fostering humanism a primary goal in aphasia group therapy?

If four or more patients with aphasia are available in one rehab setting, an aphasia group can be established. An ideal aphasic rehab program includes individual therapy supplemented by group therapy. The group typically includes four to six adult aphasia patients led by a speech-language pathologist (SLP) or another professional sensitive to the problem of aphasia. The question about fostering humanism in group therapy can be a natural outcome experienced by each member of the group. In this writer's experience, we usually had three goals in our aphasia group therapy:

- The group provides each member the opportunity to communicate with others using the best level of gesture or speech that he or she has recently experienced. The SLP reviews progress notes for each patient to be sure that patients display what "can do" words they can still say.
- The group provides for socialization. Patients react to what other group members say, or react to a statement by the SLP. Although less control of group discussion by the SLP is encouraged, the SLP makes sure that each group member is participating in the socialization.
- The aphasia group gives each member a glimpse of aphasia in other people. Patients may become aware of how other patients in the group speak with their particular type of aphasia; also, they may observe how others in the group cope with their various physical disabilities (such as hemiplegia).

In our group tale, "Honolulu Annie," less emphasis was given to our first goal of having patients use their best mode of communication (speech or gesture). Rather, group focus was on Keith with his piano playing and Annie with her wheelchair hula and singing. The others in the group were enthusiastic about her dance, giving Annie a host of automatic approval-words and musical gestures. Annie provided an excellent role model for our third group objective. She was able to perform a hula dance wearing a grass skirt while sitting in a wheelchair with only her left arm and leg able to perform. The whole group responded with gestures and humming to Keith and his piano, playing the pulsating beat of the "Hawaiian War Chant."

CHAPTER TWO

~

Tales of Dementia

While patients with aphasia have normal time and place orientation, patients with dementia experience difficulties knowing the when and where of the present and the past. The normal older population demonstrates good receptive and expressive language, demonstrating on occasion a slight immediate memory recall problem but with excellent long-term memory. In normal aging, the older person often complains of this occasional inability to remember a particular word or the name of a person or place. The dementia patient demonstrates severe retrieval problems in naming recall and in the recall of immediate and past events. The dementia patient often shows remarkably good speech and articulation skills with normal language syntax (word order) but lacks cognitive and semantic relevance. What they say may sound like normal speech and language, but the content makes little sense.

The majority of dementia patients have dementia of the Alzheimer's type. It seems to come on gradually in a linear fashion. Unlike the unilateral involvement of the brain seen in aphasia (usually left hemisphere), Alzheimer's disease involves brain structures symmetrically (both left and right brain hemispheres). The next most prevalent type of adult dementia is multi-infarct dementia, caused by the patient experiencing a series of minor strokes, with behavioral deficits developing in more of a "stair-step fashion." In multi-infarct dementia, the patient will experience more abrupt behavioral changes than the Alzheimer patient.

Occasionally, we see aphasia patients who also show developing problems of dementia. The first dementia tale, "That Would Be, Daniel R. Boone,

PhD," represents such a case. Cass, 76 years old, had been in our aphasia support group for several years at the University of Arizona before showing some of the confusions of Alzheimer's disease. The second tale, "Remember the Old Hiawatha," is about an ex-high school teacher, age 55, with Alzheimer's and with normal-sounding speech and normal grammar and syntax. He spoke in a detached manner, sounding like a monologue, lacking any voice inflection or concern for listener reaction. A university professor, his wife, and his students deal with early Alzheimer's disease in "Where Was My Mind Today?" "The Clothespin" was told by an 81-year-old woman with moderately severe Alzheimer's disease. Although she showed normal speech articulation and language syntax, what she said lacked any cognitive reality. In the final dementia tale, "The Family Picture," a speech-language pathologist hoped to orient a 74-year-old woman with Alzheimer's by working with old family photographs. The reaction he received will never be forgotten.

⁓

Tale 1: That Would Be, Daniel R. Boone, PhD

It is well recognized in medicine that a patient may have two or more diseases at the same time, related or unrelated. Cass, age 76, had two independent diseases: aphasia from a stroke followed by dementia. Some years prior to our first meeting, Cass had had a stroke that left her with severe semantic aphasia. She struggled to find proper words but physically had normal arm and leg motor functions. As she fought to find her words, she developed a perseverative phrase, "that would be," which prefaced almost everything she attempted to say. More recently, she developed a second disease, Alzheimer's, and experienced the early symptoms of confusion specific to time and place. We do not often see patients with aphasia who then develop dementia. Her tale is an interesting one.

At 72, Cass had a stroke that caused aphasia from which she made almost no speech recovery in the ensuing four years. She said "that would be" as her primary spoken response in almost any situation. However, after joining our aphasia support group at the University of Arizona and working directly with me, she modified her "that would be" by adding my complete name and degree to the utterance. Whenever she talked, she would smile and say, "That would be, Daniel R. Boone, PhD."

This response proved to be a continuous problem for me. After her dementia took over, Cass used to leave her apartment and walk to the university campus, quickly becoming lost among the countless number of students and myriad of offices and buildings. As Cass wandered lost on campus, people would react to her "That would be, Daniel R. Boone, PhD" by promptly looking for this PhD in the university directory. Subsequently, they would either walk her to my office or call me. More often than not, this necessitated me or an associate to drive her home.

As her dementia worsened, we were forced to drop her from the aphasia support group. However, this did not end my contact with Cass; in fact, our visits increased. She soon began walking within a few miles from her apartment, asking people she met on the street, "That would be, Daniel R. Boone, PhD?" with the tone of a question in her voice. At almost any time of the day or night, I would receive a phone call from an unknown person saying that a nice woman was lost and was looking for a "Doctor Boone." Once it became apparent to her relatives and neighbors that she was no longer able to live unattended (by accident and confusion, she had started two stove fires in her apartment), she was moved into a nursing care facility.

Fortunately for me, in time my name dropped out of Cass's perseverative speech pattern. If she did say it, personnel realized that my name was about all she could say and did not take her words as a literal request for my presence.

～

Tale 2: Remember the Old *Hiawatha*?

It is not unusual among dementia patients to find people who speak with great clarity about events from their remote past but are unable to recall anything about what just happened. Long-term memory may be excellent while short-term memory may be wholly lacking. Tom was such a patient. A former high school teacher, at age 55 he was diagnosed with Alzheimer's disease—unusual, because the onset of Alzheimer's disease often begins in patients considerably older than Tom.

In order to establish rapport with Tom and to provide some indication of his orientation to time and place, I asked him, "Do you still live in Tucson?" His reply prompted this detailed narrative of an incident he had experienced as a boy:

I came here from Illinois. I was raised in Deerfield, a good drive north of Chicago. The Willmans lived across the road and you had to cross through their apple orchard, if you remember, to reach the railway tracks and then walk a half a mile after that. I used to go through there, usually picking an apple, even though old lady Willman didn't like it, about once a week on my way to see the *Hiawatha*. You may remember the old *Hiawatha*? She used to come roaring through Deerfield out of Chicago on her way to Minneapolis-St. Paul. She was the flagship of the old Milwaukee Line. She was painted orange with a red stripe and, boy, could she travel. Used to come through there about sixty miles an hour. I can remember my mama telling me, "Don't get too near the tracks, Tommy, it's going over a mile a minute and it might suck you in as it's going by." But I knew that train would never hurt me. I remember her like it was yesterday, all golden, and one of the first streamliners they ever made. You could wave to the people in her cars and every now and then, one of them would wave back. There was always somebody in the last car who'd wave at you, almost as if the train was telling you "hello." One time no one waved, and I remember the *Hiawatha* tooting back at me as she went down the track to Waukegan. It was like she was apologizing for the folks in her that couldn't take the time to wave back at me. They don't make trains like the *Hiawatha* anymore. You had to tramp through the Willman's apples to get to the tracks, but the *Hiawatha* would always pay you back with a nice hello when you got there. The *Hiawatha*, do you remember her?

In later observation of Tom, I found that he often repeated the Hiawatha story to anyone who seemed to want to listen to him. He spoke with clear speech, but his voice appeared a bit higher in pitch than normal and without any kind of word inflection. He seemed unaware of his listener's response, most of the time giving a non-interactive monologue. About a half hour after our first meeting, I talked with him again. He appeared to have no recognition of me as someone who had just been with him. He greeted me with, "Do you remember the old *Hiawatha*?"

～

Tale 3: Where Was My Mind Today?

The typical older voice patient may have several competing medical, physical, or mental problems that may interfere with what we try to accomplish in voice therapy. Dr. Sam, a 64-year-old professor in the Department of Geosciences, was such an example. In the beginning of his voice problem, he had experienced some throat discomfort and noticeable voice hoarseness after lecturing for several hours to successive classes. On laryngeal examination, he was found to have "a normal larynx," and the subsequent voice evaluation identified a moderate problem of vocal hyperfunction. He was working too hard to speak. Early in voice therapy we had good luck producing greater relaxation and better breath support, and softening his way of speaking. After two weeks of twice-weekly voice therapy sessions, he missed two successive appointments. When asked about the absences, he could only say that he had forgotten about the appointments.

After missing three out of four more subsequent appointments, he apologized again for not writing down the appointment times and dates. In the fifth week, he came to the clinic with his wife, Cora, who told us confidentially that in recent months her husband had experienced a series of forgotten events. She related that one time Dr. Sam had presented the wrong lecture to a large class of undergraduates in an introductory geology class. What he started to present with detailed slides was an advanced lecture for a graduate seminar. He was embarrassed by his mistake as the students left the classroom early. Dr. Sam went back to his office and scribbled a note to himself, "Where was my mind today?" A few students even reported the inappropriate lecture to the college dean. Cora told us that his mental confusions had become more public and far more serious than any other problem he had recently experienced, such as his hoarseness.

We realized that his mental confusions relative to time and place had become his primary problem. Voice therapy was no longer appropriate. His wife reported that on several occasions he had become lost driving home from the university, a route he had routinely driven for over twenty years. She also described his crying frustration after he discovered he had lost his boxed collection of rare rock samples that he had collected over a lifetime. He wondered if he had accidentally "thrown it away." His biggest upset was the day he mistakenly deleted from his computer many pages of manuscript he had been working on for months.

Dr. Sam tried to keep his geology teaching load. In his office, he kept several calendars with explanatory notes telling him where to go, at what time to be there, and what to do after he got there. He appeared normal in both his speech and use of language. His voice seemed to no longer be a problem. The departmental secretary did what he could to minimize the professor's confusions. While most students seemed to accept his confusions and recognize his superior professional knowledge, a few had fun exaggerating the situation and laughing at his mistakes. His colleagues recognized his mental changes and did what they could in the beginning to keep him oriented to his teaching tasks. As his confusions continued to increase, however, he was finally diagnosed as having beginning stages of Alzheimer's disease. Before the end of the semester, he was forced to take a permanent early retirement.

During the early stages of Alzheimer's disease, casual speaking ability often appears normal, particularly specific to word choice and grammar. Lapses of content adequacy may occur, but the good speaking ability can often mask the patient's occasional mental shortcomings. Alzheimer patients who are individuals in authority and verbal positions (such as professors, lawyers, managers) in the beginning may be able to hide some of their mental confusions. These early confusions seem inconsistent with the patient's lifetime history of punctuality and appropriateness. In the beginning, a patient like Dr. Sam will attempt to keep his orientation by calendar self-notes. When such patients miss appointments or become confused as to where they should be, the patient and family will make excuses, which in the beginning are accepted by others.

After the early stages of the disease, when the patient becomes less aware of the world around him, the suffering of Alzheimer's disease transfers from the patient to the spouse and family. Over the last five years we have kept close contact with the professor's wife, Cora, and through talking with her have watched the progression of his dementia. In the early stages of the disease, she did what she could do to "cover" for her husband's confusions. For the first two years after his diagnosis of Alzheimer's, Cora and other family members did everything possible to keep him within their home. The need for increasing nursing care and his increasing demands for attention (often punctuated by useless arguments) forced Cora to require outside help. Finally, her case worker at a regional center on aging recommended that he be placed in a nursing care facility with other dementia patients. Such a place was found not too far from the family home.

Cora continued to make twice-weekly visits to see him, despite her gradual realization that he no longer recognized her. It always saddens me when I remember what she said at our last visit together: "When you folks worked on his voice, he made such an improvement. When he became so confused, I had hoped there would also be possible some successful treatment. But with this Alzheimer's thing, the one you knew and loved just slowly disappears on you."

I wish we could have done more. Dr. Sam recently died from an infection, unrelated to his Alzheimer's disease.

〜

Tale 4: The Clothespin

For many years, we studied the verbal abilities of patients with dementia at the University of Arizona. In general, we found that patients with dementia could speak surprisingly well. While the content of what they said may not have much meaning, the way they said it (sounds of speech, grammar, vocabulary) often sounded like that of a person with normal functioning intelligence. Mary, age 81, with moderately severe Alzheimer's disease, illustrates the contrast in demonstrating normal grammar and vocabulary but not making much sense to her listeners.

As part of our battery of tests for measuring speech and language in dementia patients, we included a task of naming objects followed by a request to tell us what the objects were used for. The patient was shown five objects, one at a time, and asked to name each one and tell us something about it. Mary was presented with a clothespin, and I asked her, "What is this?"

Holding the clothespin in her right hand, she turned it over several times so that she could examine it closely, and then said, "This, of course, is just a wood thickness, and then they have the wood itself. And we could pinch it which years ago would have been a horrible looking thing, wouldn't it? And here we have it where the wood would be."

Interrupting her, I asked again, "What is it?"

"Well, some years ago and for so many times you used it for a clothespin. This is what started it and to have it. It might get here and here and here, but it never got in this way. Likewise, they thought that they would, but because it became larger and was part of the picture, people liked it. It took over. That's all it was. Then we had something else with it."

Attempting to move on to naming the next object, I took the clothespin back and said, "So, it's a clothespin, right?"

She smiled and added, "The clothespin had its way and we'd never got too far without it. Whenever we needed it, it was around us. It was going to be something, if it had its way. And then stopped it all after finding it was a clothespin."

This elaborate answer when asked to identify an object is a typical response of a moderately severe dementia patient on a naming task. Grammar, vocabulary, and word order are relatively normal. The extensive elaboration, however, carries little or no meaning. On our five-item naming test, the typical dementia patient seems unable to give a one-word naming response. Although they may say the word in their elaborate reply, they seem to show almost no awareness of listener response. A wife commenting on her husband's dementia and difficulty in naming things stated, "He always seems to be forced to keep raving about the object, talking on and on about it, completely unaware that he is making no sense to me." Specific naming in dementia is often a difficult task.

～

Tale 5: The Family Picture

Pearl, 74 years old, had a 20-year history of vascular hypertension with elevated cholesterol, for which medical treatment had been basically ineffective. In the 1950s and 1960s, elevated cholesterol was principally treated through dietary reduction of fats. Subsequently, in her early 70s she began to experience several small strokes. This was followed by occasional episodes of time and place confusion. In the beginning of her confusions, she was aware of her problem but unable to correct it on her own. She also began to show some confusion while dressing, such as trying to put her left foot in her right shoe. Her loving husband reported that she increasingly became emotionally labile when she found herself confused, often lashing out at those around her. Upon medical examination she was found to have "multi-infarct dementia"—deteriorating brain function resulting from a "continuous series of small vascular strokes."

In the beginning, her physical appearance stayed the same; she often looked like a proper lady presiding over tea. As her dementia worsened, her husband reported that if he left her alone in their house, she might unmake the beds, take down the drapes, and get out the luggage. She would then say with normal speech, "I think we'd better get going." Her behaviors within her home and later in the home of her daughter continued to worsen, such as emptying kitchen and bedroom drawers, and packing her own clothing into the drawers she had emptied. The family eventually realized that Pearl had to be cared for outside the home in a nursing care facility.

Pearl's two adult children and her husband all took an active role in seeing that her care was good in the understaffed nursing facility. As the dementia increased, her behaviors became worse. She was observed several times by visiting members of her family walking naked down the halls, dropping into the rooms of other dementia patients to give afternoon greetings. Her need to undress herself and pile her clothes on her bed required continued monitoring by nursing staff. After six months in the nursing home, she began to dig and scratch out the grout between the tiles in her bathroom, placing the grout in her mouth, then chewing and swallowing it. She was even observed scratching out tile grout in other patients' bathrooms.

Within two years of the onset of her dementia, she could no longer recognize family members when they came to visit her. Her son, a doctoral-level speech-language pathologist (SLP), attempted to provide her with some mental focus by reviewing old pictures of family members with her. He selected a picture of his four children and placed it in front of both of them on a table. He kept his mother's attention by speaking in a louder voice, pointing to each child by name. Pearl seemed to be looking as she talked a bit in a normal voice about "nothing." She gave no evidence of picture recognition.

Finally, as a closing gesture, Pearl's son said, "OK, Mom, let me get you a glass of water." He got up from the table, went to the sink in the room, and filled a paper cup with water. When he returned, the family picture was no longer on the table. He could see in Pearl's open mouth that she was chewing it and had already swallowed two-thirds of it. The son watched in disbelief as his mother ate their family picture.

Fortunately for Pearl and her family, the dementia that had taken over her person had a quick ending. About three years after onset, her grout-eating behavior caused a massive internal hemorrhage, leading to her sudden death. The SLP son was always fascinated by the incongruity between his mother's severe cognitive decline and her continuing abilities to speak with articulation clarity and normal grammar and syntax. This personal experience with his mother's dementia, together with his professional career investigating aphasia and providing language service for people with aphasia, led to years of published dementia and language studies at the University of Arizona. I am this SLP. Pearl was my mother.

⁓

Looking Back at Our People with Dementia

These few stories can tell us something about dementia. We can see early beginnings of dementia and how it progressively worsens. Looking back at the dementia stories of our five patients, we have developed five questions that a reader might ask to learn more about dementia:

- Does keeping a daily calendar of events help the person who is beginning to experience dementia symptoms?
- Why do most people with dementia usually speak with normal language rhythms?
- As the severity of dementia increases, do most patients become less aware of their problem?
- Does Alzheimer's disease usually develop in a gradual, linear way?
- How do family members cope with the person with advanced dementia who no longer recognizes them?

Five Questions about Dementia

Does keeping a daily calendar of events help the person who is beginning to experience dementia symptoms?

One of the early symptoms of beginning dementia, either of the Alzheimer's or multi-infarct types, is some confusion of time and place. The patient typically begins a day not knowing what day it is or not knowing if there are any planned activities for that day. Dr. Sam recognized his need for a calendar with written times for everything he planned to do each day. He found that he had difficulty remembering things that were spoken to him; oral spoken messages needed to be written down. He ended up with three calendars: one for his pocket, one for his desk, and a large one hanging on the wall above his desk. He even reminded himself of needed preparation for lectures to be given the next day. Dr. Sam fought his increasing confusions by developing a written daily plan listing time and events; he then transferred these daily events to his desk calendar. His heavy use of calendar-reminders helped him remember things he needed to do early in his fight with dementia; in time, they were no longer effective.

Pearl would ask her husband each morning what day of the week it was. He would point to the wall calendar hanging above the phone in the kitchen. If there were events to do that day, such as a doctor's appointment, he had printed in large letters the event and time for that particular day. For some appointments, he asked Pearl to enter them on the wall calendar. When she completed the Sudoku puzzle in the morning paper, her husband would often ask her to look up the date posted on the top of the page. If the wall calendar listed a specific time to be somewhere, they found it useful to mark in red ink the time when they should start getting ready to leave the house to allow ample time for the appointment. Pearl's husband found it useful to have large clocks in the bedroom, the TV room, and the kitchen, three places in the home where Pearl spent time. With monitoring by both the calendar and the clock, Pearl functioned at home surprisingly well in the early months of her developing multi-infarct dementia.

Cass lived alone in a small apartment in a county retirement building. Early after the onset of her confusions, her social worker visited Cass in her apartment and brought a large digital clock to use in her kitchen. She also hung a large daily calendar in the kitchen and attempted to help Cass learn to use it. It appears that Cass was unable to profit from self-monitoring events on an event-calendar; her dementia had already become too severe.

Why do most people with dementia usually speak with normal language rhythms?

When listeners converse with the typical patient with dementia, they may be surprised to hear the patient's speech patterns sounding very much like their own. The rhythm or melody of the conversational voice may sound normal. Even the perseverative utterance, "That would be, Daniel R. Boone, PhD," by Cass would be spoken with normal inflection.

In dementia, linguistic knowledge for speaking is still there: Sequence of noun-verb words, correct verb tense, and modifiers like adjectives and adverbs are still in the right place in phrases or sentences. The problem is word selection and loss of meaning. The voicing patterns of a lifetime are still there, too; the sound of the voice and the melody of the spoken words (prosody) have meaning. For patients with dementia, the sound of their voices continues to show the emotions they may be feeling, such as happiness, anger, sadness, surprise, and so forth.

In our "Tales of Dementia," Cass, Dr. Sam, and Pearl seemed to have patterns of voicing similar to how they had spoken for a lifetime. Not so for Tom and Mary. Tom spoke in a slightly higher-pitched voice in his monologues about the *Hiawatha*, speaking with no pauses or pitch changes. Once he started talking, he seemed to be unaware that he had a listener. For Mary, when I handed her a clothespin, she turned it over in her hands, placing it closer to her eyes, and began describing it in a "tender" voice. She spoke in a slightly higher pitch, more slowly, and conveyed to me in her prosodic voice changes the emotion of caring and loving.

In a summary answer to the question, it appears that prosody, or the melody, of a language has its beginning roots in the first year of life. As a baby hears the parent language spoken, he hears the prosodic melody of that language before he knows the meaning of the words. As he acquires his vocabulary, his early spoken phases and sentences are said with the prosody of that particular language. This distinctive melody for each spoken language lasts for a lifetime, with only slight changes occurring in some people with dementia.

As the severity of dementia increases, do most patients become less aware of their problem?

The typical person experiencing the early symptoms of dementia may begin by searching for answers. Early word- or name-finding lapses might be accepted as the typical word-finding problem reported by many older people. These age-related lapses are often minimized by using calendar-reminders as discussed in answering a previous question. What separates memory confusions in normal aging from immediate memory loss in early dementia? The normal aged person still has normal awareness of time and place. The person with beginning dementia has increasing time and place confusions.

Both Dr. Sam and Pearl had early awareness of their confusions. Dr. Sam took an active role in minimizing his problems by initiating detailed notes on daily calendars specific to the "what, where, and when" of the activities for each day. By doing this, Dr. Sam was able to hide his time and place confusions from his university colleagues and students for many months. On the other hand, Pearl complained to her family about her memory confusions from the very beginning. She complained about her memory loss of newly acquired information. She withdrew from social interactions with longtime friends and preferred being alone with her crossword and Sudoku puzzles. By creating event calendars in the home, her husband provided time and place structure so she could continue to participate in some events outside the home.

For the typical patient with a developing dementia, there comes a time when the patient is no longer aware of his or her confusions. Patient care is now wholly the responsibility of the family or care center. We never saw the beginning of the dementia for Cass, Tom, and Mary; by the time we evaluated them, their dementias were firmly established. However, with Dr. Sam and Pearl, we witnessed their early concern about memory function disappear as the dementia increased. While we could view this as a welcome relief for the patient, the transfer of concern was now with the spouse and family.

Does Alzheimer's disease usually develop in a gradual, linear way?

As we read in our individual tales, four of our patients had Alzheimer's disease: Cass, Tom, Dr. Sam, and Mary. Pearl's developing confusions were the result of multi-infarct dementia (often called vascular dementia) caused by a series of small strokes. In Alzheimer's, there is a slow, continuous loss of memory; in contrast, the memory loss in multi-infarct dementia is characterized by abrupt, stair-step changes. (In chapter 6, we will further contrast the gradual onset versus the abrupt changes of the two dementias.)

Cass presented a confusing diagnosis. We saw her first in our aphasia clinic after she had experienced the abrupt onset of a stroke. All she could say was "that would be," communicating only by the inflections of her voice. We followed her for two years, working with graduate students under my direction and supervision, but she made no progress in her speaking ability. We were able to follow her gradual memory loss and increasing time and place confusion. It became obvious that Cass had two overlapping diseases: (1) a stroke causing aphasia and (2) a developing memory loss from Alzheimer's disease.

In our medical clinic, we evaluated both Tom and Mary for their memory loss. Each had had a previous diagnosis two or more years earlier of Alzheimer's disease. We were able to follow them over several years in an ongoing dementia study, finding slight increases of memory loss in both Tom and Mary. The gradual continuing deterioration of mental function was well documented by Dr. Sam and his wife, Cora, in his early struggle with Alzheimer's disease.

With multi-infarct dementia, the mental changes in Pearl were much more abrupt. Her husband and family observed that what she could do well (such as dressing herself) on one day, she might be unable to do at all on the succeeding day. Pearl's dementia from beginning to end lasted only three years; her sudden death ended her family's concern over her increasing memory loss.

How do family members cope with the person with advanced dementia who no longer recognizes them?

It is a difficult time for the families of dementia patients when the patient no longer recognizes them. Usually, by the time lack of such recognition occurs, the patient requires an increased amount of care, often more mentally and physically, than the family can provide. In the story, "Where Was My Mind Today," we read how Cora (Dr. Sam's wife) did everything she could do to keep her husband at home. After two years, Cora and her family were forced to place him in a care facility. She went to see him twice weekly despite her gradual realization that he no longer seemed to know who she was.

Pearl's family had a similar experience of lack of recognition as to who they were. In the story, "The Family Picture," her son hoped to help his mother recognize family members by showing her a family picture, pointing to each person and naming them in a louder voice. Not only did Pearl not show recognition, but while her son was distracted, she ate the picture.

Inability to recognize one's spouse and other close family members usually occurs some months after the patient first needed more personal care. This lack of family member recognition more often shows itself for the first time after the patient has been away from home, living in a care facility. This lack of recognition of spouse and close family members usually occurs toward the end of the continuing dementia.

CHAPTER THREE

~

Tales of Neurogenic Disorders

We have looked at aphasia and dementia with a mixture of laughter and tears. We now look at neurological disorders and their particular impact on patients and the people around them. A particular disease or trauma to the brain or spinal column is classified as a neurological disorder. The term *neurogenic* applies to the cause of a clinical behavior that has its origins from a particular neurological disorder.

One of the speech-language pathologists' (SLP) tasks with neurogenic communication patients is to search for residual abilities that have not been altered by the faulty neurological system. Also, there is usually a functional overlay to various sensory or motor disabilities experienced by the neu-rologically impaired person. That is, patients with the same disorder will function or respond in different ways from one another, depending on such variables as cognitive ability, personality, motivation, family reactions, living situations, and/or availability of professional services. While habilitation of neurogenic communication disorders cannot usually alter the cause or main-tenance of the problem, overall communication abilities can often be raised by the SLP reducing distractions, finding optimum response situations, and listening/watching closely to the needs of the person.

Although we'll keep our descriptions of various neurogenic disorders as free of medical jargon as possible, we will define a few conditions that affect communication. Unlike the speech and language variations heard in aphasia, *dysarthria* is a motor speech problem. The speech of the patient with dysar-thria is compromised in different ways: slurred articulation, altered speaking

35

rate, with voice quality and resonance distortions. Dysarthria is a frequent consequence of such disorders as stroke, cerebral palsy, brain injury, Parkinson's disease, multiple sclerosis, amyotrophic lateral sclerosis, and many other lesser-known degenerative diseases of the nervous system. Dysarthria may be caused in part by paresis (muscle weakness) or paralysis (absent or spastic muscle action). Also, lack of central muscle coordination plus respiratory difficulties are often contributing factors to the motor speech problem.

Apraxia is the inability to perform a purposeful motor act on command, but being able to perform the same motor task spontaneously (when not asked to do so.) Oral apraxia, a motor disorder involving primarily the lips, jaw movement, and the tongue, can exist isolated or found in combination with expressive aphasia or with some dysarthria. For example, the patient with oral apraxia may be unable upon request to blow on an unlit match; however, when the match is lit, the patient can blow out the burning match immediately. The marked distinction between the inability to perform an intentional motor act (blowing on the unlit match) contrasted with normal function for the same act done spontaneously (blowing on the flame) is always an amazing clinical phenomenon to observe. Gait apraxia is equally amazing. Gait apraxia is often seen in association with Parkinson's disease, where the patient will have difficulty walking through an open door, but have far less difficulty walking across a room. In some neuropathological conditions, the patient may have apraxia for raising his arm upon request, but have no difficulty raising it when a ball is thrown for him to catch. We will read later about a patient who had no trouble sitting automatically in a chair, but when asked to "sit down," he demonstrated an apraxia for sitting (he could not initiate the series of movements required to sit when asked to do so).

In this neurogenic section, we look at some real-life situations experienced by eight neurogenic patients and the reactions of the people around them. I have used the first tale, "The Examination," in training medical and SLP students throughout my career. In the mid-1960s, I was the state consultant for cerebral palsy while teaching at the University of Kansas Medical Center. This young man with cerebral palsy taught me and the students by my side not to let a patient's diagnostic label mask our ability to hear how and what the patient has to say.

The second tale, "See You Tomorrow, Bonnie," describes the interaction between a teenaged female with cerebral palsy and her SLP, perhaps providing insight as to the danger of SLPs getting too close psychologically to their patients. "Come to Bed, Frank" is the story of a fireman who acquired an apraxia for sitting. The patient, Frank, recovered totally from his apraxia symptoms (caused by a massive smoke inhalation–induced encephalopathy), and looks back with humor at his temporary inability to sit on command when asked to do so by another person.

The physical ravages experienced by many people who suffer from degenerative neurological diseases are often overwhelming. One such person, a 52-year-old former tennis professional with amyotrophic lateral sclerosis (ALS), comments on his growing physical problems in "I Am a Prisoner." In "Winning the Fight Over Parkinson's," a 54-year-old woman experiences dramatic speech success in decreasing her Parkinson's symptoms by using intention speech therapy. We never know what to expect in the responses of the young traumatically brain-injured patient who we meet in "Dr. Lincoln." A 44-year-old woman, who had suffered severe neuromuscular problems interfering with normal speech for a lifetime, is able to experience success when shooting a modified bow and arrow in "The 'Robin Hood.'" Gait apraxia, an inability to initiate walking steps, is described in "Here Comes the Elevator" by a woman with Parkinson's. After receiving an effective medication (dopamine) regimen, she was able to reduce her gait apraxia and eventually could laugh at her memories of when she was unable to step into an elevator.

⌒

Tale 1: The Examination

The speech-language pathologist learns early in clinical work not to prejudge patient performance by the label the patient is carrying. I learned this best while examining patients, ranging in age from 1 to 20, with cerebral palsy at the University of Kansas Medical Center. I functioned as the state consultant for cerebral palsy, testing patients once a year who were brought in from around the state of Kansas. I evaluated these young patients, assisted by a few speech pathology graduate students. Each patient was tested for hearing, self-feeding skills, oral mechanism function, speech articulation competence, and expressive conversational language. I am sure that none of the students, nor I, will ever forget Ed, age 20, diagnosed as having "severe athetoid cerebral palsy."

As part of an orthopedic cerebral palsy clinic, we set up an evaluation booth that included an audiometer, a tape recorder, and our speech-language testing materials. Prior to each patient's arrival, the students and I selected the materials and tests we wanted to administer consistent with the patient's diagnosis. Athetoid patients like Ed generally displayed flailing arm movements that interfered with fine oral movements, often making clear speech impossible to produce. We planned to look closely at how Ed was able to coordinate his breath with his mouth movements for speech; this would include assessing his jaw control, tongue dexterity, and facial-lip movements. If we could understand his speech, we planned to administer an articulation test that would differentiate the sounds he *could* say from those he could not produce correctly. Also, patients with athetoid cerebral palsy often demonstrate trouble understanding the speech of others, so we had a detailed test ready that would pinpoint his language comprehension. If he could speak several words clearly enough, we planned to assess his expressive language functions.

One of the graduate students wheeled Ed in his wheelchair into the examining room. As I looked up from my desk, I saw a young man writhing in his chair, with his head twisted to one side and his arms flailing in the air above his head. His legs were locked across one another above his ankles. Such writhing movements quickly confirmed in my mind that his "severe athetoid" diagnosis was correct. Nodding at the students to begin the examination, I moved over to the patient and introduced myself. Thinking he might be hard of hearing, I said in a louder than normal voice, "I'm Doctor Boone, good morning."

Ed quickly looked up at me and said with normal speech, "Tell me, Doctor, what does this communication examination entail?"

Startled by his clear, intelligent question, I mumbled back, "Well, in your case, I don't think it will entail very much."

His appearance and his diagnostic label had not told us that he was a junior at the University of Kansas. All we tested was his hearing that day, as he demonstrated better speech and language than most of his examiners.

⌒

Tale 2: See You Tomorrow, Bonnie

Early in my doctoral training program in the early 1950s, I lived on the grounds and worked at Highland View Hospital in Cleveland. Half of the patient population was an elderly custodial population; the remaining half of the patient population (about 175 people) consisted of neurogenic patients participating in an active rehabilitation program. Three speech-language pathologists (SLPs) provided the speech-language services (evaluation and therapy) that were needed. While the majority of rehabilitation patients were post-stroke, we had a surprising number of multiple sclerosis (MS), Parkinson's disease (PD), and amyotrophic lateral sclerosis (ALS) patients, and some with traumatic head or spinal cord injuries.

We also had a special population of 15 cerebral palsy (CP) patients, ranging from 12 to 35 years old, all of whom received intensive medical and rehabilitation care. The CP patients were part of a long-term study to see if intensive rehabilitation (physical and occupational therapy, vocational training, and speech pathology services) would help for each individual to function more independently in the future. Of some interest to the curious reader, the eight CP patients who with rehabilitation therapies improved the most, reaching some degree of functional independence, were those who demonstrated less motor involvement in the beginning of their rehab program. Several of the severe patients, often with combined spasticity/athetoid muscle problems, showed almost no improvement.

This talking tale is about the 15th patient in the long-term study. Her name was Bonnie. She was 14 years old with moderately severe athetoid cerebral palsy. Besides her flailing arms and legs, she had developed a severe spinal scoliosis (her thoracic spine curved severely to the right). Consequently, as she sat in her wheelchair, her upper body, neck, and head leaned moderately to her right.

Bonnie worked with me in individual speech therapy sessions for three 30-minute sessions a week. We had a dual therapy focus, working on improving chewing/swallowing (improving vertical posturing and developing better mouth closure) and improving speech intelligibility (matching auditory modeling with her own productions). She also participated twice weekly with five or six other patients in a CP support group (a favorite task was trying to resist reacting with startle responses to sudden auditory and visual stimuli). There was also time for spontaneous conversation, laughter, and occasional tears.

Bonnie had a teenage "crush" on this clinician, particularly because her favorite singer was Pat Boone. Not only was my name "Boone," but I had met and talked with Pat Boone on a plane trip to Chicago. I was a young, newly married man, and Bonnie took extra interest in meeting my wife (a PT in our program) and our baby girl. My attempts to change her SLP to a female colleague on our staff proved to be very upsetting to Bonnie, so I stayed with her.

The assistant medical physiatrist on our CP project became increasingly concerned about the growing severity of Bonnie's spinal scoliosis. At one of our staff conferences, it was decided that Bonnie required orthopedic surgical intervention to correct her spinal deformity. Some concern was raised about her athetoid flailing movements presenting a real obstacle to the healing process after surgery. To prevent such movements of her body, it was decided Bonnie would have to wear a body cast post-surgically for six to eight weeks to stabilize her torso. Some staff raised concerns that she might not be able to tolerate wearing such a rigid post-operative cast, since for a lifetime she had had continuous flailing movements of her arms and legs, which seemed to accentuate the bending of her torso. The orthopedic surgeon flatly stated that he would not be able to correct the curve in her spine unless she wore the body cast for at least six weeks after the surgery.

Therefore, a trial body cast was placed around her six weeks before the scheduled surgery. If she could not tolerate it, the cast would be removed and the planned surgery would be canceled. Bonnie tolerated the cast well for six weeks. Inhibiting her uncontrolled movements actually improved our work with her in both feeding and speaking. We talked freely about the coming operation day when the cast would be removed, the surgery completed, and a new body cast put in place. When that final cast was removed, she would then be able to sit and even walk in an upright position, as she said, "like everyone else."

I joined other staff members in explaining to Bonnie and her family how much better she would be able to do things after the surgery. The surgery was scheduled for a Monday morning. I remember well my visit to Bonnie in her hospital bed early Sunday evening with her single parent, her mother, sitting next to her. I remember kissing her on the forehead and Bonnie kissing me on the cheek. I remember telling her goodbye with a little assurance when I said, "See you tomorrow, Bonnie, after the operation."

Bonnie died the next morning in the operating room.

Apparently, Bonnie died as a reaction to the anesthetic. Her weeks in the body cast with the enforced lack of body movement before the procedure had weakened her total system. I had become very fond of Bonnie as a person. I questioned my medical colleagues after her death about the necessity of restricting motor movements in a young patient with cerebral palsy, who had spent her short lifetime with hyperactive motor activity, twisting her torso and flailing her extremities.

Her sudden death bothered me. More than a clinician working on swallowing and talking, I had become a close friend. I also learned a career lesson: never become too close emotionally with a patient. With any kind of negative outcome, such closeness can really take a toll on the clinician.

〰

Tale 3: Come to Bed, Frank

Some patients after brain damage have problems of apraxia. As mentioned in the introduction to this chapter, apraxia is the inability to do things on purpose (like blowing on an unlit match) contrasted with normal motor movements for automatic functions (like blowing out a lit match as it is brought closer to one's mouth). In apraxia, there is a dramatic difference between normal function for automatic situations and the complete inability to perform "on purpose," or volitional movements. Some apraxia patients have problems moving their mouths; some cannot take a step if told to do so. Frank, age 37, was a victim of an unusual apraxia, an inability to sit down if told to do so by someone else. He could sit down normally if he were not asked to do so.

Frank was an athletic fireman, 37 years old, in excellent health until the day he inhaled a large amount of toxic smoke while fighting a plastics fire. The continuous exposure to these fumes resulted in an "encephalopathy" that affected parts of his brain, resulting in (among other symptoms) an apraxia for sitting down.

Referred to my office in a rehabilitation hospital for a speech evaluation, I observed that Frank had some difficulty sitting down. When the office receptionist told Frank to sit down in the waiting room, he replied, "Oh, I wish you hadn't said that." He consequently remained standing until I came out and ushered him into my office. We talked casually while walking into my office, and I motioned for him to sit down. Instead of sitting in the chair in front of my desk, he stood behind it and then circled around it several times, saying, "Oh, I wish you hadn't pointed to the chair." If someone told him to sit or even pointed to a sitting place, he could not sequence the correct motor movements to sit down. After bending his knees several times and hopping to the front of the chair, he was finally able to lower his body into the seat.

Once comfortably seated, Frank told me, "It's the damnedest thing, Doc. Since my accident, I can't sit down if someone tells me to do it. If I walk in a room on my own and see a chair or a bed, I can sit down with no problem." He was describing the classic symptoms of apraxia, the inability to do with intention what he can do automatically.

Frank and I became good friends during his hospital stay. He volunteered to help us with a much-needed service: pushing wheelchair patients from their wards to our speech clinic and back to their rooms when the speech therapy appointment was over. He had no problem walking or taking patients to the clinic. At times, when accompanying patients, he would come into the waiting room, sit down (fortunately, no one told him to), and have a cup of coffee with patients while they waited for their appointments.

After being an inpatient in our rehabilitation hospital for four weeks, I participated with other professionals in Frank's discharge planning conference. His wife also attended the conference. She told us about the problems she had with Frank's sitting when he first came home on a weekend pass. Apparently, after they both got dressed for bed, she got in bed first. As Frank approached the bed, she made the mistake of saying, "Come to bed, Frank." Immediately, Frank began bending down in a tight circle trying to sit, as he cried out, "Oh, I wish you hadn't said that." According to his wife, his shifting, circling movements continued until he accidentally fell into bed.

There are specific and focal movements that we all do to accomplish a motor task, such as sitting. For most of us, there is not much difference between the automatic execution of the task or deliberately doing the same movement. Frank's inability to sit on purpose (with preservation of normal automatic ability to sit) was an apraxia for sitting, a rare symptom of brain damage caused by his extensive inhalation of toxic smoke. Fortunately, within a few months after the onset of his problem, Frank made a complete recovery (no more sitting apraxia), and eventually he was able to go back to working as a fireman.

～

Tale 4: I Am a Prisoner

About a month before I evaluated Mike in our hospital department, I had talked to him casually at our mutual tennis club about a frontal lisp he felt that he was developing. Mike was 51 years old, a tennis pro who had enjoyed a lifetime of robust health. At one time, Mike had coached me on my tennis game, and despite my limited progress we had remained good friends. However, in the last few months, he had lost his balance on the tennis courts and had even fallen twice. Seeking medical help, as part of a total medical evaluation, he was referred for speech-language services regarding his increasing problem producing sibilant sounds like /s/ and /z/.

Audiological testing found Mike to have basically normal hearing with a slight high-frequency loss not atypical for his age of 51 years. Language testing was basically confined to conversation about tennis and world events, with Mike displaying normal comprehension and language. His connected speech, however, did show a slight sibilant /s/ and /z/ distortion. On a peripheral oral evaluation, he showed two abnormal tongue findings: (1) When asked to stick out his tongue and hold it out, the tongue showed fasciculation (a traveling wave across the tongue surface); and (2) he had some difficulty when asked to elevate his tongue tip up behind his upper incisors, as if he were making the /t/ sound. Particularly disturbing to me was the observation of tongue muscle fasciculation, where several fibers of the tongue muscle are twitching simultaneously, producing the wave-like movement on the surface of the protruded tongue. Our observations suggested a possible muscle problem of neurogenic origin, and he was referred for a neurological examination.

We did not see Mike again in our department for several months. He continued to work as a tennis pro, but was experiencing increasing problems walking and running on the tennis courts. Further neurological observation and testing finally came up with the diagnosis of amyotrophic lateral sclerosis (ALS), often called Lou Gehrig's disease. The cause of ALS is unknown. It involves nerve tracts in the lower part of the brain and upper spinal column and is classified as a lower motor neuron disease. No medical or surgical treatment is available to prevent the progression of the disease. There is gradual deterioration of muscle function in both legs and arms, and involvement of tongue and throat muscles involved with speech, swallowing, and throat clearing.

About four months after his ALS diagnosis, Mike experienced enough leg muscle deterioration that he was no longer able to work teaching tennis. He spent a few hours a day in the pro shop, selling tennis goods and restringing racquets (his upper extremities remained functional). There was some increased slurring of his speech, and he was forced to speak slower than normal, probably related in part to slower tongue movements.

We initiated speech therapy when he began to experience some difficulty feeding himself. He began to experience some choking when swallowing, particularly when drinking fluids. We worked with him on head posture, mouth closure, and attempting to increase the rate of tongue movements. Language function remained normal. We worked with him to increase speech intelligibility, making special efforts to produce tongue movements (accuracy and speed) for such sounds as /k, g, t, d/. He was a fighter for improvement and was always able to temporarily improve some function. Mike came to see us intermittently over a two-year period, whenever his speech or swallowing would worsen.

Although Mike's speech could still be understood, he needed our help for back throat activities such as swallowing and clearing his throat. We worked closely with him related to clearing out throat mucus, coughing, and the pooling of mucus-fluids in the back of his throat and under his tongue, requiring the use of a syringe when needed to suction out the fluids he couldn't clear on his own. His overall leg and body control worsened, and he was forced to use a wheelchair. I remember one of our last visits with Mike, now only 52 years old, when he told us, "I am a prisoner of my own body."

Mike described his plight well, and the unfortunate progression of degenerative nervous system diseases like ALS. Speech therapy, like other rehabilitation programs, can help the patient maximally use all remaining systems that have not been involved by the disease process. It cannot prevent further disease progression. Mike and his family had almost three years after the diagnosis of ALS to make as much out of life as possible. Mike remained cheerful and thoughtful of those around him, his family and church friends, tennis buddies, and the team of medical workers who provided him the care he needed. Counseling with clergy was a great help to Mike and members of his family. Similar to other patients toward the terminal days inflicted by ALS, Mike began to breathe in (aspirate) the fluids accumulating in his throat, eventually dying from the collected fluids in his lungs. Appreciating his valiant fight for life, I will always remember him and his haunting words, "I am a prisoner of my own body."

～

Tale 5: Winning the Fight Over Parkinson's

Over the past few years, we have observed an apparent increase of patients with Parkinson's disease (PD). As the disease progresses, increasing speech and voice symptoms are often lessened by the services of a trained speech-language pathologist (SLP). About the time the Parkinson's patient experiences difficulties walking, he or she may be experiencing difficulties speaking, with voice loudness problems. A typical complaint of PD patients is that they are continually asked to repeat louder what they have just said.

Normal speech is a fast automatic neuromotor event. We don't think about where we are placing our tongue to make the speech sounds nor do we have any awareness of what our vocal folds are doing. Automatic motor movements, like walking and talking, are compromised in PD; these movements are controlled by a collection of nuclei deep in the brain, known as the basal ganglia. The neurons in the basal ganglia communicate with one another by a neurotransmitter fluid called dopamine. Parkinson's disease is the result of absent or low dopamine levels. Successful treatment, therefore, requires a dopamine stimulant, as well as physical therapy and speech pathology services.

Phyllis, 62, possibly experienced her first PD symptoms five years ago while singing in her church choir. When she was standing, holding her choir book in her left hand, she could feel a tremor in her dangling right hand; however, when she reached across to turn the page, the right-hand tremor would disappear. She subsequently experienced slight difficulty walking and some increasing difficulty being understood when she was speaking. She consulted a neurologist, and after extensive testing, this was her diagnosis: "This cooperative, intelligent woman is showing early signs of Parkinson's disease. She should begin a regimen of L-dopa, coupled with physical and speech therapy." The hand tremor at rest (non-intention), which ceases with intentional movement, is a classic symptom of PD, as were her changes in gait and some slurring of speech.

For the first three years after her diagnosis, Phyllis did well taking her medications. However, she elected to have little physical therapy. She consulted with several SLPs about her speech, and she received minimal speech pathology services at two different speech clinics. About two years later, while attending a Parkinson's support group, she saw a video about SPEAK OUT!, a speech rehabilitation program that is partially based on a therapy program for PD developed by me in the 1950s. It was based on my observation that when the PD patient did things with intent, performance improved. For example, when asked to count forward from 1 to 15 (an automatic motor movement), the patient's speech was slurred and voice was barely audible. In contrast, when counting backward from 15 to 1 (more intentional), speech and voice sounded more normal.

Phyllis entered the SPEAK OUT! program, which for her required 14 individual therapy sessions and five once-weekly group therapy sessions. When working on breath control, she was given time targets, such as prolonging the saying of "ah" for exactly ten seconds. Or she worked on voice glides and short speech phrases, keeping her voice at target intensity levels (monitored on a sound-level meter at 80 dB). The target intensity levels were primarily imposed to keep intention as part of the loudness task. She did very well at home in daily practice using both timing and loudness targets to maintain deliberate or intentional speech. It was in the weekly follow-up group sessions that Phyllis really found herself. Her friendly, outgoing personality, coupled with her excellent speech, made her a popular group member.

We have made several videos asking Phyllis to speak about using intent and deliberation as a primary way for the Parkinson's patient to maintain good speech. When the person with PD goes back to automatic speech, his or her speech deteriorates. Therefore, unlike what the SLP usually does at the conclusion of speech therapy for other problems, which is encourage automatic speech/voice production, the best speech/voice in PD is maintained by continued use of intention.

~

Tale 6: Dr. Lincoln

This brief anecdote is included as a tale to add some levity and needed balance to this neurogenic section. Josh was a 22-year-old head trauma patient who had received four weeks of speech-language therapy. After a dramatic recovery from most of his disabilities, he was scheduled for a hospital discharge planning conference.

Following ten days in a coma after an automobile accident–induced head injury, Josh, upon awakening, showed some motor deficits in his left arm and leg with left facial muscle weakness. He showed some cognitive deficits, inappropriate use of language, and a mild dysphagia (problems in swallowing). About four weeks after the accident, he had made significant improvement and was scheduled to return home to live with his mother and younger brother. Any further rehabilitation therapy could be provided to him as an outpatient.

Josh was able to walk well with a cane. His mother had come to his ward, and they walked together to our clinic waiting room. I came into the waiting room and announced his name. They both stood up as I extended my hand to greet them, and Josh said to his mother, "Mom, this is the man I've been working with on my speech. I want you to meet Dr. Abraham Lincoln."

Before I could correct his name selection, his mother joined in, "So glad to meet you, Dr. Lincoln."

I answered, "Well, Josh has the right idea about my having a famous American name. But it isn't Lincoln." I paused as I added, "I am Daniel Boone."

We all shared some embarrassed laughter as we went to the seminar room for our part in the discharge planning conference.

For me, questions about my ancestry or some teasing remark about my name have been common occurrences for a lifetime (I had two sons and wisely did not pass on the name "Daniel Boone"). However, this was the first time that anyone had ever mistakenly substituted my name for another historical fig-ure. In Josh's case, it was consistent with problems he was having in specific word recall. He knew I had the name of a famous American historical figure. He just could not remember which one.

⌒

Tale 7: The "Robin Hood"

My first view of Alice over five years ago was behind a one-way observation window in our university speech clinic. She and her mother had returned to the clinic to see if once again things could be done to improve her speech. Clinic records over many years showed that Alice had Friedreich's ataxia, a disease that shows up at pre-adolescence and remains for a lifetime. Typical signs are scoliosis, inward turning of joints, and difficulty making any kind of deliberate muscle movement. Alice began to show her first symptoms at age 9, and now, at age 44, her overall symptoms were more severe, with her speech almost impossible to understand.

She lived with her mother, who was also her caregiver and sole means of support. She was wheelchair dependent, and always walking closely beside her chair was Cassie, her loyal yellow Labrador dog, who for several years had been an important part of Alice's life. Our speech evaluation focused on her poor voice, which interfered with anything she wanted to say. Her voice seemed to suddenly appear, with loud gasps coming though her nose. With a little modeling of a light voice, attempting to say a few words at a time, one could understand what she was saying. We enrolled Alice in our clinic program for voice therapy, and she soon made modest but temporary improvement. Now for several years, working with the same SLP for a few weeks every month or so, she has been a willing client for our graduate stu-dents to work with in developing their voice therapy clinical skills.

Alice recently had a life-changing experience that came out of her work with her SLP. When talking about sports in a therapy session, Alice wist-fully noted that she would have liked archery if she had the muscle ability to hold a bow and pull back on an arrow. Immediately after the therapy session, unbeknownst to Alice and her mother, we contacted our local rod and gun club, who referred us to Arnold, a local young man who was a national archery champion. After observing Alice in therapy through an observation window, Arnold was confident that if Alice had the eyesight to calculate distance through a scope, he could adapt an archery shoot that she would be able to use.

Alice was invited the next week to practice archery with Arnold at his local archery range. She arrived with her mother and Cassie (her dog) leashed to her chair, but she was quite apprehensive over her ability to shoot an arrow. But Arnold had rigged a crossbar contraption that allowed Alice to peer through a scope, make minor adjustments to the bow resting on a bed of sandbags, and then pull the crossbow trigger with her right index finger. She hit a bull's-eye at 20 yards, then 30, then 50. Her second time shooting, she shot an arrow that split her first arrow sitting on the target. This phenomenon, explained Arnold, is called a "Robin Hood," making Alice a member of that most exclusive archery club. With this pronouncement, Alice lifted her gaze from the sight and announced with a grin, "After all these years, I can finally say I am good at something!" Cassie, still standing next to the wheelchair, wagged her tail in agreement.

⌣

Tale 8: Here Comes the Elevator

Rose, 52, had a five-year history of progressive motor involvement from Parkinson's disease. Her main concern was a severe gait apraxia, which at times made it impossible for her to initiate walking forward. As she attempted to walk when asked to do so, she would take many short steps in place but could not step forward. Similarly, when asked to walk through a doorway, she often could not initiate the steps necessary to walk through it. Her speech had a slight dysarthria characterized by rapid articulation and a very light voice. She also had non-intention hand tremor; at rest, her hands would be tremulous, but when asked to touch her nose, she could do so quickly without tremor.

This particular tale occurred in the mid-1950s when Rose was a patient active in our speech pathology program in a rehabilitation hospital.

While Rose was in our rehabilitation program, she received speech therapy every day at 11:30 in the morning. Within the therapy session, we focused on talking louder, even encouraging her to yell speech responses. When speaking with such deliberate intention (speaking inappropriately louder), her speech was much more normal in rhythm and clarity of articulation. Besides providing her speech therapy, it became my job every noon to walk beside her as she returned to her ward for lunch. The speech therapy offices were on the fourth floor and her ward was on the third, necessitating that we walk the length of two corridors and then negotiate the elevator. Once we got started, Rose could walk the hallway with no difficulty, shuffling ahead with small steps but in a steady gait. She would shuffle down the fourth-floor hallways holding my arm until we reached the elevator. We stopped and I pushed the down-button. Rose and I then stood waiting, and we could see the numbers flash by above the door as the elevator approached our floor. About one floor ahead of the elevator's arrival, Rose began to shuffle her feet in place, moving neither forward nor backward. Bothered for some time by her gait apraxia, she knew that she was going to have trouble stepping into the elevator when the door quickly opened.

The elevator door would open, and four or five people riding up or down would look out at us as Rose shuffled in place, unable to move toward the door. 1 took her arm, saying, "Come on, Rose, let's get on." Quickly she would answer in her rapid speech, "I would if I could, but I can't, so I can't move in." As she shuffled in place, I said to the people in the elevator, "You folks go on, we'll catch the next one."

As the elevator door closed, I pushed the down-button again. We repeated this procedure several times, each time hoping to board the elevator, but with no luck. Then I remembered that if we could set up an automatic walking situation, it would be easier for her to walk into the elevator. So I said to her, "Rose, this is how we can get on the elevator. First of all, we'll stand back further from the elevator so we'll have more room to walk. As we look up and see that the car is coming to our floor, I'll start tapping you on the arm and we'll match each tap by counting aloud together. We'll start our count just before the elevator gets here and begin walking forward toward the door. Then when the door opens, we can just sail in as we are counting 1-2-3-4-5-6."

Our "entry" plan worked. We counted as we walked and skipped rapidly into the elevator, often startling the other passengers with our unique entrance.

Our problems, however, did not end with our boarding the car. We remembered that the same sudden door opening problem would make it difficult to get *out* of the elevator. We soon found that we were lacking adequate walking distance to "count-walk" our way out of the elevator. We had to walk across the width of the elevator car. The door would open at the third floor, but it opened and closed so abruptly that we couldn't easily use our counting system. I can remember astonished staff and friends looking in on us as the door opened at various floors. I would playfully yell out, "We're taking an elevator tour ride today."

Rose and I decided that as the elevator approached the third floor, we would begin our sidewise count-walk early enough so that when the door opened, we would be scooting through. The first step was "one," the second step was "two," and so forth. It often took us a few rides down and a few rides up before we had the timing perfected so that our walk from the back of the elevator was uninterrupted in rhythm and timed exactly with the opening of the door. As the door opened, we were through it.

Gait apraxia is always more severe the more focal the situation, such as walking through a door the second it opens. It would have been easier for us to push Rose back to her room in a wheelchair, but part of the philosophy of the rehabilitation hospital was to encourage as much walking as possible. I am sure that many hospital staff and certainly most visitors were startled by our unorthodox style of entering and exiting the elevator.

Walking through doorways, particularly those with automatic opening doors, is particularly difficult for the rare patient with gait apraxia. Usually such an apraxia is only found in occasional patients with Parkinson's disease. Despite her attempts to diminish the gait problem in her physical therapy sessions, Rose had experienced little success. Things improved for her when a successful medication regimen (elevating combinations of dopamine, norepinephrine, and serotonin) was finally established. The last time I saw Rose, she was experiencing less gait apraxia, and she also had improved the quality of her speech and diminished some of her non-intention hand tremor. She also laughingly reminded me, "Remember when the two of us couldn't get in the elevator? And when we got in, we sure as hell couldn't get out!" I remembered it well.

~

Looking Back at Our People with Neurogenic Disorders

As the brief stories of the eight people with neurogenic disorders illustrate, there is a great diversity of disorders producing a variety of symptoms. Such diversity makes any one answer to the following five common questions difficult to respond to with one global answer. Instead, we will look back at what was known about each of our eight people and how their particular neurogenic disorder would influence their probable answers to the questions. The questions are:

- **Do most patients with neurogenic disorders possess normal intelligence?**
- **Is motor disability using arms and legs a prominent symptom of neurogenic disorders?**

- Can the dysarthrias experienced by this population be helped by speech therapy?
- Do most patients with neurogenic problems (like MS, ALS, CP, or Parkinson's) have normal hearing and understanding of spoken and written language?
- How does apraxia affect the patient's motor responses?

All eight of our patients were referred to us by physicians in a medical setting. Their medical records usually included psychological test results and hearing screening. Most patients had been active in both physical and occupational therapies. Most of them had been seen by other SLPs before we had the privilege of working with each of them.

Five Questions on Neurogenic Disorders

Do most patients with neurogenic disorders possess normal intelligence?

A common experience by patients with severe motor problems of speech (dysarthria) is that they are often viewed by listeners as having limited cognitive abilities or intelligence. People speak slower and louder to them in the hope of improving their comprehension of what is being said. Ed, now 20, with moderately severe spastic athetoid cerebral palsy, said that as a boy he wished that people would have spoken to him with a normal rate and loudness. Phyllis noted that when her Parkinson's got bad, almost everyone said something like "What?" in a louder voice every time she spoke. She said that because of her poor speech, people thought "I was dumb." While Alice had difficulty responding on a psychologist's test because of severe motor problems in both speaking and pointing, the psychologist concluded that "her reactions to questions indicated probable normal intelligence."

Other than Ed and Bonnie, whose problems of cerebral palsy (CP) were observed at birth, our other six people acquired a neurogenic disorder in childhood or later in life. As we will see later, in chapter 6, many literature studies support the observation that in the overall CP population there is an approximate 60 percent prevalence of reduced intelligence. In contrast, Ed's quickness of word indicated probable normal intelligence.

Both Frank (sitting apraxia) and Josh (word-searching problem) had some temporary reduction in cognitive function; however, follow-up contact with each of them indicated total recovery. It appears from clinical research literature that cognitive abilities are often reduced in neurogenic diseases. We shall cite in chapter 6 various studies that have presented data on intelligence for each of three major acquired neurogenic diseases (ALS, MS, PD);

a combined summary of these studies found a mild prevalence of reduced intelligence among patients with these diseases. Three of our people (Mike, ALS; Phyllis, PD; Rose, PD) displayed relatively normal cognitive ability and therefore do not fit into the summary category of reduced intelligence for their particular diseases.

It would appear that the people and their tales in this chapter cannot validly answer the question of normal intelligence in patients with acquired neurogenic disorders. Family members and friends may believe that the patient's slower motor responses represent some reduction of intelligence rather than the result of reduced motor function. Intelligence testing avoids measuring intelligence by the quickness of response in this population.

Is motor disability using arms and legs a prominent symptom of neurogenic disorders?

Many people who acquire some form of neurological insult experience no overt sensory or motor symptoms of their arms and legs. In our tales, only Frank exhibited a lack of motor involvement of his extremities. Frank had such good motor control of his arms and legs that he was able to help other patients transfer to wheelchairs and to offer his arm and hand to those who needed some help in ambulation. His apraxia for sitting only showed when he was asked to sit. Josh early in his treatment showed left hemiplegia with severe perceptual and linguistic problems. When we last saw Josh, despite continued mild left-sided weakness, he appeared almost robust in his fast walking and skipping in the physical therapy gym.

The absence or presence of physical symptoms is related to the site and extent of the brain lesion. We remember in chapter 1 that most of our people with aphasia had unilateral left hemisphere lesions resulting in right-sided weakness. In chapter 2, our dementia patients had a progressive bilateral loss of brain function with some reduction of bilateral fine-motor skills. In this chapter, our seven other people besides Frank had various motor symptoms using their arms and legs.

Our most severely involved person with motor disability was Alice with Friedreich's ataxia. Since adolescence and up to when we saw her, she had almost no functional use of her arms and legs. On some days, she had almost no speech. At other times, she could say a few sentences that others could understand. Both Ed and Bonnie with athetoid cerebral palsy experienced flailing extremities with various amounts of spasticity. Our two people with Parkinson's, Phyllis and Rose, each experienced some non-intention tremor in their hands: at rest, their hands would shake; if they reached for something, the tremor would cease. Mike with ALS experienced a worsening of motor symptoms as the disease progressed; his facial, palatal, and throat muscles became most involved.

Can the dysarthrias experienced by this population be helped by speech therapy?

As a speech-language pathologist (SLP) with a career of many decades, I could give a strong "yes" to the question. However, a more convincing affirmative could come from our patients with some kind of neurogenic problem. Ed would be a strong example. Even with severe cerebral palsy, with a lifetime of speech therapy he developed good functional speech. By age 20, his superior intellect and strong motivation made it possible for Ed to attend the University of Kansas. The focus of therapy for Bonnie was on increasing her ability to chew and swallow, with less emphasis on speech clarity.

Both Rose and Phyllis profited from speech pathology services. Rose received speech therapy centered on increasing respiratory control to give her a much-needed louder voice. Comparison of speech-voice recordings taken of Rose before and after therapy showed the positive effects of speech therapy. Phyllis was part of a Speak Out! program that used the effects of intention on both gait and other movements, with focus given to deliberation of speech. Taking the automatic way of speaking away and replacing it with deliberation gave her more articulate speech and a louder voice. Mike was able to prolong his life by the speech intervention he received specific to chewing and swallowing. He worked closely with his SLP in his attempts to swallow, learning successfully to use a syringe to remove pooled liquids in the bottom of his throat.

The positive effects of speech therapy for some neurogenic problems are more difficult to quantify. The archery achievement award given to Alice had an obvious psychological impact on her. Josh initially had severe motor-perceptual problems after his traumatic brain injury. He displayed some language difficulties with a problem of word retrieval. Our use of a modified word association program along with some word-game apps seemed to contribute to his observable improvement in conversational fluency. We have never seen another "sitting apraxia" like we saw in Frank, and we probably never will in the future.

Do most patients with neurogenic problems (like MS, ALS, CP, or Parkinson's) have normal hearing and understanding of spoken and written language?

Among our eight patients with neurogenic disorders, only Bonnie had a mixed conductive-sensorineural hearing loss. She tested with an average 30 dB threshold across the speech-recognition frequencies; however, this mild loss did not appear to handicap Bonnie, as she responded to spoken directions. Our two Parkinson's patients, Phyllis and Rose, were found on hearing tests to have mild high-frequency losses, a typical hearing response for people in their 50s. The literature suggests no typical pattern of hearing loss for patients with Parkinson's disease. The other five people in our neurogenic tales had normal hearing in both ears.

In answer to the latter part of the question, each of our eight people were able to follow and understand spoken instructions. Any slowness of response was related to hand or oral muscular incoordination or weakness. Reading function was tested only to third-grade comprehension levels. Only Alice had difficulty reading.

The person who acquires some type of neurogenic disorder does not usually have the severe auditory and visual problems of language experienced by the many children with developmental and language learning delays. The reader must remember that the population with acquired cerebral disorders is uniquely different from the infant and young child who has yet to experience normal language. In adults who develop a neurogenic disorder, their relatively normal hearing and visual systems are still there.

How does apraxia affect the patient's motor responses?

In apraxia, there is a marked difference between the patient's automatic and deliberate motor responses. We saw this dramatically when Frank could sit down automatically when he didn't think about it, in contrast to his inability to sit when directed to do so. The SLP confronts oral apraxia in both children and adults. In children with developmental aphasia, learning to speak is sometimes complicated by oral apraxia. In acquired aphasia, the patient has had existing speech before the causative accident or stroke. This existing speech can still be used automatically and spontaneously, even in the form of perseverations. We saw this in chapter 1 with Mary Lou's continuous response of "damn shoes." Her inability to initiate any other speech may have been related to a persistent oral verbal apraxia. In the treatment of expressive aphasia with oral apraxia, the SLP searches with the patient to find words and phrases he or she can still say. Early treatment hopes to expand on the patient saying these automatic utterances with less demand for struggling to say something new. The aphasic patient's oral muscles are still normal and capable of producing normal speech; however, if oral apraxia is also present, it may prevent the initiation of saying any words with intention.

We saw the struggle Rose experienced with her problem of gait apraxia. Most people with advanced Parkinson's disease walk with an altered gait, characterized by stepping forward with smaller steps. While Rose walked with a small-step shuffle, she had the additional problem of gait apraxia. She could not get her leg muscles to walk forward when approaching a door. The more focal the door opening, like boarding an elevator, the more severe the influence of gait apraxia. Our successful ability to access and leave an elevator required the use of automatic counting from 1 to 10, coupled with taking a step with each number.

For those patients who experience apraxia as part of their neurogenic disease, there is a marked difference between automatic and intentional motor responses. The goal of therapy for different forms of apraxia is to increase overall muscle function by using more automatic motor and speech systems.

CHAPTER FOUR

~

Tales of Voice Disorders

In the normal speaking population, we take our voices for granted. Our breathing is adequate to support a normal voice, which always seems to be there for us with adequate loudness, appropriate pitch, and a relatively normal voice quality. The sound of the voice (phonation) is produced by actual vibration of the two vocal folds (also called vocal cords), generated by the outgoing air stream passing between the approximated folds, setting them into vibration. The vibration produces the sound of voice. This is why normal voicing is so dependent on adequate and normal respiration. Severe breathing difficulties can make normal voice production impossible. In voice therapy, voice is often improved by better coordination of breathing with the timing of one's speech.

The pitch range of the voice is related to the overall size, thickness, and tension of the vocal folds. Infants and young children have higher-pitched voices related to the relative smallness of their vocal folds. With physical maturity, the larynx and airway become larger and the voice deepens. The pitch of the speaking voice and of the singing voice is directly related to the size and thickness of the vibrating vocal folds. Changes of pitch are related to tension changes in the folds. As the vocal folds shorten, they increase in thickness, producing a lower pitch. Voice pitch continues to get higher as the vocal folds are stretched thinner, increasing their tension and producing a faster vibration or higher pitch. With laryngeal growth at the time of puberty, the female voice pitch drops about half an octave, while the male voice drops a full octave or more.

The resonance of the voice (quality, nasality) is determined by the relative openness and relaxation of the throat, mouth, and nasal passages. Resonance disturbances are often related to infections, allergies, and throat-nasal tissue problems.

A voice disorder can be caused by problems of respiration and/or phonation and/or resonance. The ear-nose-throat physician (ENT, or otolaryngologist) and the voice clinician (usually a speech-language pathologist [SLP]) work closely together in the management of children and adults with voice disorders.

Most voice disorders are classified by the ENT or SLP as either functional or organic in origin. A voice problem that is functional in causation is a poor voice produced by a normal mechanism in a faulty manner. For example, a young high school cheerleader uses his or her voice without adequate breath support and produces a strain on the vocal folds, resulting in a hoarse voice. With proper voice training, normal vocal mechanisms usually can produce a normal voice. An organic voice disorder may be heard in a hoarse, strained voice that is produced by physically altered mechanisms. For example, a vocal fold with a cyst on it will produce a faulty voice. The cyst hinders the normal vibration of the involved vocal fold, hindering the quality of voice. After removal of the cyst by the ENT surgeon, with some vocal training following the surgery, the patient may experience a normal voice again. In many voice cases, there is a mixture of functional and organic components. This is why anyone with a voice disorder should have a thorough diagnostic workup before receiving any kind of voice therapy.

As a voice clinician, it has been my clinical experience that many voice patients with functional voice problems often possess personalities that are a bit "friendly hyper." The patients are extroverted, laugh a lot, and are somewhat happy personalities, but also often somewhat controlling of the people around them. Their voice problems are often related to excessive muscle tension and continual voice usage. In contrast (and this could be a faulty observation), the personality patterns of patients with an organic cause of their voice problem seem to fit in well with the general population. Most voice patients, regardless of the cause of their voice problem, are desperate for help and will follow closely the voice regimens developed by their SLP to help them achieve a normal voice.

In the tale, "Signal Light Practice," I follow the self-practice antics of an attorney with a functional voice problem. The importance of one's voice pitch level in establishing gender identification on the telephone is told in the second voice disorder tale, "I Am My Wife." The danger of putting a person on "voice rest" is then described in a tale of a seven-year-old girl who lost her voice completely in "No Talking for Ten Days." A woman who had her larynx totally removed because of laryngeal cancer tells us that the worst problem she experienced with no voice was being unable to voice her emotions, as told in "I Can't Laugh or Cry." With voice therapy, the coach in "Coaching Basketball Without a Voice" found his voice again. In "Piano Lessons with Chopin," we laugh with an older woman with a wandering personality who could never get around to talking about her voice problem. A 44-year-old female executive in "A Little Voice" describes the difficulty she had expressing authoritative decisions with her "tiny voice." As some laryngectomy patients continue to smoke after total surgical removal of the larynx, a 60-year-old maître d' tells us about his smoking problem in "A Smoky Good Evening." These are but a few talking tales with laughter and tears that I pulled from the files of many voice patients over the years. For most voice problems, the presenting problem can be minimized, no longer offering humor or sadness to the patient's observers and listeners.

⌒

Tale 1: Signal Light Practice

Tom, a 64-year-old attorney, continually developed some hoarseness at the end of the day after having used his voice all day in various professional settings. An otolaryngological examination confirmed that he was experiencing some mild vocal fold swelling, "probably secondary to misuse of his voice." Our clinical voice evaluation found that Tom utilized very little breath support for what he wanted to say, demonstrated some neck and jaw tension, and generally spoke with an abrupt, hard glottal attack. A striking observation found that Tom hardly opened his mouth when he spoke, almost speaking through clenched teeth. To illustrate his closed-mouth talking, we asked him in jest, "Have you ever been a ventriloquist?" When he laughingly said "no" to the question, he got the message of the need to open his mouth more as we replied, "Well, you could be good at it, as you rarely open your mouth much when you speak."

Among the various voice exercises we asked Tom to practice was to open his mouth more as he spoke. We used an old chewing therapy method, where the patient pretends he is chewing up a stack of several crackers with an exaggerated mouth opening while repeating some kind of phrase. We provided him with a nonsense word model, AHLAMETERAH, which he was to say while performing the exaggerated chewing. The sounds of the model enabled him to speak the "word" with an open mouth. His other voice exercises were more conventional, often using some kind of auditory playback equipment.

Because practicing exaggerated chewing makes the patient look ridiculous, it is best done alone. We often recommend chewing practice while driving the car, as it provides the patient with an excellent private practice time and place without observers. One must continue repeating the exaggerated movement until it becomes more automatic, resulting in a more conventional mouth movement of lips and jaw while speaking.

Tom did a lot of driving in his work, giving him ample time for chewing practice. He was even able to have fun with the practice. He told us of driving his car while chewing with a wide-open mouth, and one day stopping at a signal light, waiting for the signal to turn green. Adjacent to his car on the right was another waiting driver who had glanced over at Tom with a startled look and kept staring at him until the light changed to green, when he yelled across to Tom, "I don't know what you're on, fellow, but be careful!"

When Tom told us this story the next week in therapy, we knew that the message of opening one's mouth more when speaking was a talking rule that he would never forget. Working on better breath control, speaking with an easy onset of words, and letting his voice resonate more fully with a more open mouth all seemed to fuse together, giving Tom a normal voice throughout the day, with a total elimination of voice strain.

～

Tale 2: I Am My Wife

One of the more disturbing voice problems one may encounter is speaking at an inappropriate pitch level, with a voice either too low or too high. A man might sound like a woman or a woman might sound like a man. Obviously, this kind of gender confusion can be at its worst while speaking on the telephone. We judge the gender of the people with whom we are speaking, in part, by their voices. Although there is sometimes a physical cause of an excessively low or high voice pitch, it is often something one has learned to do that could be corrected by voice therapy. Thornton was a 51-year-old swimming pool maintenance man who came into the voice clinic with an inappropriately high-pitched voice.

The referring letter said that while Thornton had always had a higher voice, it became even higher after he inhaled excessive chlorine gas in a swimming pool servicing accident. Four weeks after the incident, he sought help for his voice. When asked at the first interview why he had come to see us, he answered, "I am my wife on the phone and people are beginning to think that she is me." He went on to elaborate that when he answered the phone, his high-pitched voice confused his listeners into thinking he was his wife. He felt, also, that his wife, who had a low-pitched voice, was often mistaken for him. Although they laughed at the gender confusion between them and their phone listeners, it was becoming a serious problem for them socially. He wanted help.

A few sessions of voice therapy helped to lower his speaking voice about two full musical notes, although his voice was still well within the adult female range of speaking voices. To sound more masculine in his speech, particularly on the phone, he was encouraged to drop his pitch inflection toward the end of an utterance. In general, men tend to lower their voices at the end of a sentence while women often have a slight rising pitch-inflection. Also, speaking with a crisper, more abrupt speaking manner is heard by listeners as more masculine than feminine. By incorporating both these speaking styles, dropping inflection and speaking with more abrupt word pronunciation, Thornton was able to help his listeners on the phone know that they were speaking to a man. His pitch level, for reasons unknown, never returned to pre-accident levels.

The voice pitch that an adult uses plays a primary role in gender identification, particularly on the telephone where the speaker cannot be seen. Other masculine speaking traits, such as dropping inflection and speaking with abruptness can be added to the phone voice to aid in gender identification. Besides voice pitch and pitch inflections, the loudness of voice and the rate of speech contribute to gender identification. Communication research between the sexes has found in general that men speak a bit louder with a faster rate of speech than women do. When the speaker can be seen in face-to-face situations, masculine body posture and gestures can also help in accentuating one's gender.

⌣

Tale 3: No Talking for Ten Days

Penny, at age seven, did a lot of yelling and a fair amount of crying. By the end of her first year in school in the 1960s, she began to experience severe voice hoarseness. Her parents took her to a Cleveland ENT, who found that

Penny had "bilateral vocal nodules." Vocal nodules form on the middle of the vibrating muscle of the vocal folds, caused by continuous voice misuse (yelling, screaming, crying, and talking loudly). Nodules are usually found similar in size, somewhat symmetrical, on both vocal folds. Today it is felt that the best way to get rid of these vocal masses is by counseling and voice therapy designed to minimize the causative vocal misuse. In the early 1960s, however, nodules were more commonly removed surgically, followed by up to two weeks of complete voice rest in which the bilateral surgical sites would heal.

The nodules, one on each vocal fold, were successfully removed for Penny by surgery. To promote healing, the surgeon instructed the parents to do everything they could to keep Penny quiet (no talking, no crying) for up to two weeks. The parents answered the doctor's request by saying that they would do what they could, but since Penny had always been very active vocally, the "voice rest" requirement would be difficult to enforce. The doctor was very good with Penny in explaining the need for voice rest, and as she left his office, he remarked again, "No talking now for ten days."

About two weeks after surgery, the parents brought Penny back for her postoperative examination. They reported that Penny had been very good about not making any vocal noises. In fact, they had not heard her voice in the two weeks since the surgery. On examination, the ENT doctor reported that she had very good vocal fold healing and said, "Go ahead and talk, Penny, all you want." The child smiled back, grabbed the doctor's coat, and whispered to him, "I can't find my voice anymore." The doctor replied, "Let me help you," and he made several suggestions, but Penny could only shake her head without making any voice. The family returned home, and no matter what they did, the child could not produce voice.

One of the dangers of putting a voice patient on voice rest is that the patient may find other ways to communicate, such as Penny had, by gestures and whispers, without the need for voicing. She could only speak in a whisper. Three to four weeks after the nodule surgery, she still had no voice. The ENT surgeon then referred her to our university clinic with this referral notation: "This 7-yr old child had bilateral vocal nodules removed and after a brief voice rest, she has refused to try to talk."

We found Penny to be very cooperative during our testing and therapy, even though her first voicing attempts met with failure. We found that there was some truth to her mother's statement that "Penny seems to have forgotten how to talk." We countered, "She seems eager to talk, but can only do so in a whisper." Her voiceless speech was categorized as functional aphonia.

We were able to confirm early in our voice evaluation that the child demonstrated a normal cough when asked to do so.

Coughing demonstrates that the vocal folds are not paralyzed and can physically come together. When an individual coughs, the vocal folds are brought firmly together and then suddenly parted by an explosive outgoing breath. A firm cough tells the clinician two things: (1) The vocal folds are not paralyzed, as they are brought together with firm muscle contractions; and (2) the coughing sound can be extended through voice therapy into normal voice. This confirmed the observation that Penny was experiencing a functional aphonia, a voiceless condition not related to organic factors such as paralysis.

I explained to Penny that sometimes when people stopped using their voices after surgery, they had some trouble "getting their voice started again." Voice was kind of like an engine, "it needed a starter to get it going." I was planting for her the "seed" that total voice return would be possible because we knew how to get it started. We were soon able to get Penny to make a light coughing sound, after which I commented, "There, I can hear the vocal cords coming together again. Did you hear that noise when you coughed? That sound was your voice coming off of your vocal cords."

We then showed Penny how to extend a light phonation after the cough. Instead of coughing abruptly, we held onto the cough with an extended voice. We then introduced "cough-onnnnne," a method for hanging onto voice after the cough by introducing the word "one," prolonging its production with a light voice. Penny was thrilled with the voicing of her first word in many weeks. We tempered our reaction to her voice success (it's easy to scare the phonation away by clinician overreaction). We spent about ten minutes producing about a dozen monosyllabic words that she could say after the light cough. By the end of our first session, Penny was able to use a light voice without need of the facilitating cough, the "cough starter." We kept our voice list short, to about 15 words, demonstrating to her mother how easily Penny could say them.

We terminated the session after a clinic hour, and told Penny to practice the words on the list just as we had done and to do no more than those 15. We scheduled her return clinic visit for the next day. However, Penny was so excited by her discovery of her voice that she would not stop practicing that evening. By the time she went to bed, her parents reported that Penny demonstrated a normal voice for whatever she wanted to say. She came in the next morning to our clinic a very happy girl with a normal voice. We celebrated with her, and before she left the clinic, we planted another "seed," which often helps the voice patient who may be fearful that his or her voice may be lost again: "Penny, you've found your voice again and your voice 'starter' will never, never leave you." In a nine-year follow-up for Penny's reactive aphonia after voice rest, the family reported that she never again lost her voice.

Functional aphonia is usually treated effectively by the speech-language pathologist, often requiring only a few therapy sessions. Methods for restoring phonation include the cough-extension method described for Penny, or using inhalation phonation as a method for finding voice, or asking the patient to whisper-read aloud and then introducing loud masking noises (which will often turn the whisper into actual voice). Functional aphonia usually has a very favorable outcome with restoration of normal voice.

Penny had surgical removal of bilateral vocal nodules followed by an enforced voice rest. That was 50 years ago. Today, most vocal nodule problems are successfully treated by voice therapy alone. Surgical treatment of the vocal folds is still needed, however, for such problems as vocal cysts or vocal fold webbing. Voice rest is then used post-surgically, with some voice patients experiencing difficulty retrieving normal voice after the voice rest has ended. It seems like the voice patient has "forgotten" how to phonate.

Because of this occasional problem of retrieving voice, it has been my clinical observation that complete voice rest should be avoided after most vocal fold surgery. Instead, we encourage the patient to use a light voice or a "confidential voice," the kind of voice used in a private conversational situation. Such a light voice does not seem to add any irritation to the vocal folds as they are healing after certain kinds of surgical procedures.

～

Tale 4: I Can't Laugh or Cry

Roberta, a 54-year-old black divorced mother of three teenagers, was kidded continuously about her low-pitched voice. She had for years worked in a downtown Denver coffee shop and was able to support her family from alimony monies, wages, and some very good tips. Unfortunately, she had developed a habit of smoking, consuming nearly two packs of cigarettes a day. In her busy life, she was able to balance her mothering duties with church responsibilities and her lunch and evening work as a waitress.

As her hoarse voice deepened in pitch, she also developed an annoying cough. Since waiting on tables limited her ability to cough when she wanted to do so, she did two things: She coughed as lightly as possible in public, or made frequent trips to the employees' restroom where she could cough heavily enough to clear out the offensive mucus. It was her coughing problem, not her deep voice, that forced her to seek medical attention.

The ENT found that Roberta had extensive cancer of the larynx, severe enough to require the surgical removal of her entire larynx (laryngectomy). This would require breathing through a surgically created opening in her neck (tracheostomy), plus the need for developing a new substitute voice (esophageal speech). The very day that she was told of her cancer diagnosis, Roberta vowed to quit smoking (and has never had a cigarette since). To help Roberta understand what she was facing, she had several pre-surgical visits from two women who had received the same kind of operation and had made wonderful recoveries. They each spoke to her with their new voices, describing how their family lives and work experience had continued on very well. Their inspirational stories convinced Roberta to proceed with her total laryngectomy—the total removal of her larynx, or voice box.

Roberta had a successful laryngectomy operation, followed by some radiation therapy around the operative site. The surgeon helped her develop a new substitute voice by making an opening between her windpipe and esophagus, and then inserting a small plastic tube through the opening, enabling her outgoing breath to flow into her esophagus. Once in the esophagus, this air can then escape through the esophageal sphincter, the muscle opening at the top of the esophagus. When expired air passes through this tight opening, it produces a burp sound. This is the same mechanism any person uses whenever we belch out air. In the case of the laryngectomy patient, this air-sound is used as a substitute voice. Patients who are good at using this esophageal voice can often say six or more words at a time on one continuous belching sound.

With the referral of one of the laryngectomy visitors who had visited Roberta before the operation, she began receiving voice therapy lessons with a speech-language pathologist (SLP). The SLP worked with her to increase the amount of air she could use for vibration of her esophagus. In a few sessions, she was able to say two words at a time, particularly words that began with explosive sounds like /p, b, t, d, k, g/. Roberta was determined to get back a usable voice that would enable her to return to her work as a waitress. She joked with her voice clinician that her new voice sounded more like a woman's, higher in pitch, than her old low voice.

Roberta was invited by several of her new voice friends to attend a laryngectomy support group. Every other week, a group of voice patients met for an evening of chat and coffee among themselves and family members. Roberta had always had an open, gregarious personality, and as soon as she was able to say a few words, she actively participated in group discussions.

One evening, she surprised the group when she talked about voice and emotion, saying, "Not having a voice is one thing, but the thing I miss the most with my new burp-voice is that I can't laugh or cry." She went on to say that the laughing voice and the sobbing voice just did not feel the same with her new substitute voice. She said that one way she had always coped with her family obligations without a husband on the scene was to shut her bedroom door and then lie down and cry. After sobbing a bit, she felt relieved and able to cope with the family's day-to-day problems. She missed not being able to have a normal crying voice.

Roberta went on to become one of the best esophageal speakers I ever heard in my professional experience. Like the two women who had visited her prior to her surgery, she signed on as a visitor friend to talk to new laryngeal cancer patients. She not only became a proficient speaker, but her role as a working mother was exemplary to new patients concerned for their futures after surgery. Although we never forgot her "I can't laugh or cry" comments, she learned to feel and express those emotions again. Her sensitivity to human needs after surgery made Roberta one of our most valued visitors to see new patients before receiving a laryngectomy.

⌒

Tale 5: Coaching Basketball Without a Voice

Attending an athletic event, or when actively playing sports, can be hard on the voice. Yelling loudly is encouraged in many football stadiums or basketball arenas, with the crowd encouraged to yell louder. Their loudness is shown by increasing decibel levels that change colors or light brightness displayed on large panels. Everyone is encouraged to make a lot of noise. The problem is that most people in the crowd do not know how to yell. Similarly, athletes in some sports (football, soccer) are sometimes encouraged to use an aggressive voice, which is often low-pitched and extra loud. After excessive loudness or yelling, many people experience temporary problems with their voices (hoarseness or a voice that isn't loud enough or a complete loss of voice).

Speech-language pathologists (SLPs) in community or medical clinics frequently see children and adults who develop voice problems from using too loud a voice. Children, for example, do a lot of yelling on noisy playgrounds. A politician running for office may make a series of speeches without amplification, forcing him or her to produce a loud voice, often over loud background noise. By the time the hoarse patient seeks the help of an SLP or vocal coach, he or she may have experienced voice symptoms for weeks or even months. The first step is to receive medical clearance by an ENT. Voice therapy begins by identifying the cause of the voice problem, in this case, excessive loudness. The first goal in therapy is to identify the situations that force extra loudness, and then hopefully reduce or avoid them. Patients are then evaluated as to how they produce voice at various loudness levels. Voice tests are made specific to breathing techniques, voice pitch, ease of voice production, resonance, and other behaviors the SLP may feel contribute to the faulty voice. Finally, a therapy program is developed for each person for achieving a more normal voice.

The therapy program for a hoarse voice caused by excessive loudness is two-fold: (1) reduce or eliminate the need for a loud voice; and (2) use some new methods for producing a louder voice. In the case that follows, Coach Fred, a high school basketball coach, couldn't avoid the situations that prompted him to use a loud voice, so with voice therapy, he learned to use a louder voice, and at times, he was even able to yell without hurting his voice.

Coach Fred, age 44, had been the basketball coach for the Centennial High Rams for the past 16 years. He prided himself every year for recruiting 10 to 15 strong, tall boys, and through his coaching and a favorable schedule, he won eight citywide championships. However, he had had trouble with his voice for over five years. He reported that after several hours of daily practice, yelling out to the team and demonstrating court maneuvers, he would start to have a hoarse voice. After actual games, where he had yelled instructions to the players on the court and often argued with officials, he sometimes would lose his voice completely.

Finally, upon the urging of his wife, Fred self-referred himself to our university voice clinic. We found that his hoarse voice and occasional total loss of voice were indeed the result of using a loud voice against a background of excessive noise. We recognized that we couldn't lessen the noise and the tension he experienced while coaching, but we could teach him to use a voice that would hold up under such adverse conditions. Our therapy began by learning to take in deeper breath and use it to punctuate the voice. Following demonstration, he was able to use the "barker" voice, more forward in the head with a slight tinge of nasality. By using much auditory and video feedback in therapy and self-practice, Coach Fred was able to develop and use the voice he needed in his basketball coaching.

Some people experience voice difficulties when trying to speak in difficult situations, such as against a noisy background. Coach Fred was one of those people, losing his voice in tense and noisy situations. He did not know how to yell against a noisy background. With some voice therapy, he was able to develop a compensatory voice to use in both basketball practice and game situations. This also enabled him to find and use a normal voice when he was not coaching.

∼

Tale 6: Piano Lessons with Chopin

Over the years, I have often noticed new adult voice patients express a need to validate their trust in the voice clinic that they are considering for help with their problem. They will frequently cite the referring physician's comments that coming to see us will resolve their voice problem or that this clinician "knows what he is doing." The patient wants to express his or her faith in the new voice evaluation and treatment. I will never forget one patient's comments. We'll call her Wanda, a well-dressed woman in her mid-60s. When I went to pick her up in the waiting room, she stood, extended her hand, and said, "Oh, Doctor, I'm thrilled to meet you. Having voice therapy with you is like having piano lessons with Chopin."

Her greeting was only the beginning of a most unusual clinic evaluation. The voice clinician working with adult patients will occasionally see a patient similar to Wanda, whose free-flowing personality revealed communication problems far beyond concern for a hoarse voice. Her fun, eccentric, outgoing need to talk made it difficult to conduct any kind of vocal assessment. When we counseled her that voice therapy would not be of as much help as perhaps psychological counseling would be, she embraced the idea of seeing a psychologist when she replied, "Imagine me with a few sessions with Sigmund Freud."

A glimpse or two of my voice evaluation attempts with Wanda well illustrate why voice therapy was not possible. As we walked to the clinic office, I asked her why she had come to our voice clinic to see us. She quickly answered in a loud voice, "Oh, Doctor, I've been wanting to get after my voice for months now. My bad voice is getting in the way of everything I try to do." This was one of the few mentions of her voice problem in the entire interview. She quickly provided me with a full case history, with very little questioning possible by me. What was so remarkable about her case, and the reason I have resurrected her dialogue, was the detailed narrative she provided about bizarre events in her life that seemed to have little relevance to her voice problem.

I asked her, "How does your voice get in the way of the things you want to do?"

She answered promptly, "It's the birds, Doctor, it's the birds. Some days they can't hear what I try to tell them."

After telling me that weekly she put out over ten pounds of birdseed in her backyard for "the birds of Denver," she went on to say that "some of my neighbors did not like me anymore because the birds were always flying over their properties, soiling their roofs, their sidewalks, and their driveways. The birds want to flap their wings and sing their songs of love and happiness. But so many of my neighbors would rather polish their barbecues and scrub their lounge chairs than listen to a thrasher sing." It became quickly apparent that her hobby with the birds had isolated her from her neighbors.

During our one-hour evaluation, Wanda never stopped talking. Another example of her talking can be seen in this tape-recorded segment:

"Doctor, did you ever see a robin have a convulsion?"

"No, I've never seen any kind of bird have a convulsion." I answered.

"Well, it's the pesticides, Doctor, that get to them. It hit this dear little robin one Sunday morning, and I go out to the feeder, and he's twitching there looking up at me for help. I held him and did what I could because I knew him. He'd been at our place every spring since I can remember with his whole family. But somehow he got into the neighbor's yard with all his chlordane and other killers and it got to him. I've gone up and down the street talking to the folks that live there to switch to buttermilk. You see, buttermilk is the best pesticide we have because it kills the insects and leaves the squirrels and the birds alone. My robins know that, my doves know it, but that Sunday morning one of my dearest robin friends couldn't get enough to eat at my place, so he drifted over next door or some place and ate their flower poison. By the time he got back to our sanctuary, the chlordane had hit his darling little brain and he got the convulsion. You could almost see his little brain pulsing to push out the poison. I am sorry to say, he never came out of it."

All attempts that I made to get the patient back to the issue of her voice problem were usually met with other long narratives, generally about her birds, but also about saving the rabbits and the coyotes. Problems with her voice were the least of what concerned her.

While Wanda sounded as if she had a voice problem, her overriding problem appeared to be a number of environmental concerns and problems with her neighbors. It was apparent early in our interview that voice therapy designed to curb her excessive talking would not be successful. When it was pointed out to her again that she might profit from talking with a psychologist, she seemed to accept the idea. However, follow-up with her psychologist revealed that after two sessions, Wanda had discontinued further appointments. I met her by chance at a grocery store several years later, and she voiced her concern to me that the organic foods had been contaminated. She warned me by saying something like this, "You sure don't want to buy those organic berries, Doctor. You pay more for the organic fruits, which are heavier with poisons than the regular fruits, despite the fact that the grocery people deny it." Listening to Wanda in the grocery store brought back old memories of our voice evaluation several years before.

⁓

Tale 7: A Little Voice

Catherine had worked as a manuscript reader for a major publishing house for about ten years. She had recently been appointed as a senior acquisitions editor whose frequent responsibility was meeting with various authors to discuss manuscript strategies. For a lifetime, she had been kidded by others about her baby-sounding, high-pitched voice. Finally, she came to our voice clinic wondering if voice therapy would help her develop a more professional voice to use with her author clients, both on the telephone and in face-to-face meetings. The baby-sounding voice was quickly apparent as she answered questions during the history-taking part of our evaluation. We explained to her early in our testing that the baby-sounding voice was primarily caused by placing one's tongue too far forward within the mouth.

During our voice evaluation, we were able to confirm by two ways that Catherine carried her tongue too far forward in her mouth: (1) When videotaping her mouth as she spoke, we observed a lot of forward tongue; and (2) lateral x-ray imaging confirmed excessive front-of-the-mouth tongue carriage as she spoke. We also found that her voice pitch was significantly higher (just below middle C4) than that of most women her age (G3). We scheduled her for individual voice therapy.

It did not appear that the higher voice pitch contributed much to the baby sound of her voice. Therefore, we placed therapy emphasis on what we call "voice focus," where the voice seems to have its origins and resonance focus. A normal voice sounds like it is coming from the middle-top of one's mouth, almost sounding as if it were resonating from the surface of one's tongue. We explained to Catherine that there are four main resonance deviations in voice focus: (1) too far forward, (2) excessively back in the throat, (3) down low behind the tongue in the base of the throat, or (4) a nasal focus with voice coming out of the nose. We told Catherine that in therapy we would begin by developing back throat focus, the very opposite of what she showed us when producing her baby voice. In the beginning of therapy, we practiced making the back sounds of English: /ka/ and /ga/. These two sounds are made with the tip of the tongue down in the front of the mouth with the posterior tongue body arched high up against the roof (palate) of the mouth. We used a playback solid-state recorder for her to say back sounds (/k/ and /g/) and then hear an immediate playback of what she had just said. We recorded her producing a few /k/ and /g/ sounds in a series like "kuh-kuh-kuh"—"kah-kah-kah"—"guh-guh-guh"—"gah-gah-gah." Producing these back sounds immediately got rid of her baby resonance, replacing it with full posterior resonance, which we called for her a "big voice."

Catherine was surprised and thrilled that in the first few moments of voice therapy she was able to produce and immediately hear herself producing a back voice. We cautioned her that the back voice was a "means to an end." We would use the back voice focus only temporarily. Eventually, we would work on lowering her voice pitch, but our beginning therapy would focus on producing appropriate voice focus, giving her an immediately more pleasant voice. She required practice with the back voice before we proceeded to bring the voice to a normal, more forward position. We also discussed that the "front voice" and the "back voice" were only imagery concepts, not factual absolutes; that is, voice seems to resonate more forward or backward in the mouth. Before the next therapy session, she reported back to us that she had never stopped practicing the series of /k/ and /g/ sounds.

She found driving the car a good place to practice, too, and whenever she found herself alone, she found great joy in using the back voice sounds.

In subsequent voice therapy sessions, we practiced repeating, at different loudness levels, individual /k/ and /g/ words like "comb, come, corn, gone, gun, gum." She would record her voice on a playback recorder and listen immediately on playback to her back voice productions. After 100 percent success producing back words, she advanced to reading sentences heavily loaded with /k/ and /g/ sounds. Catherine remained highly motivated in therapy and eventually had an easy time bringing her voice "more forward" to normal resonance levels. She could read aloud maintaining good resonance focus and avoiding extremes in both anterior and posterior tongue carriage. At the last therapy session, even her conversation was completely free of the baby voice that she had when she started therapy.

We have continued to talk to Catherine by phone over a number of years, and we always hear a normal voice. Catherine recently told us, "I can still remember the awful baby voice that I had. It never seemed to match the responsibilities that I had in my publishing world. I can now use my voice to serve me." Getting rid of her anterior voice focus was a wonderful example of success using symptomatic voice therapy. We ignored working only to lower her pitch and worked instead on changing her voice resonance, using excessive posterior resonance to help her eliminate excessive anterior tongue posturing, the primary cause of her little voice.

⁓

Tale 8: A Smoky Good Evening

A throat cancer patient may have to have his or her larynx (voice box) removed surgically. Such patients then develop a substitute voice either by belching up air from the esophagus, which sounds like a hoarse voice, or by placing a small electric instrument against the neck that produces a vibration that results in a mechanical voice. Such patients breathe through an opening in their neck, which permits air to flow in and out of their lungs. Unlike a normal throat that allows both air and food to pass through together before separating to either the lungs or the stomach, patients with their larynx removed (laryngectomy) have breathing and eating as separate anatomic functions. All breathing (inspiration and expiration of air) passes through the opening in the neck (tracheostomy). Whatever contents are in the mouth can be swallowed and diverted back down to the esophagus and then into the stomach.

Harvey had been a maître d' for many years at one of Cleveland's finest restaurants. Even after he had throat cancer necessitating a laryngectomy followed by voice training, he went back to work with his new voice and resumed greeting patrons at the door when they entered the restaurant.

After his operation, he still liked to smoke, but now found conventional smoking almost impossible. He'd either have to place the cigarette directly in the neck opening (which he found most unpleasant) or derive a little tobacco taste by attempting to inhale through his lips. Since his mouth was surgically disconnected from his airway and lungs, the smoke that gathered in his mouth could not be inhaled and would often be swallowed down into his stomach.

One of Harvey's favorite stories to tell after his laryngectomy was of a night at work when he forgot to empty his stomach of smoke. On a break from his maître d' duties, he went to the employees lounge to enjoy a menthol cigarette. He had found that menthol cigarettes felt better in the back of his throat than conventional cigarettes. He smoked the cigarette down, swallowing much of its smoke into his stomach. Usually after smoking this way, he remembered to belch up the smoke before he began talking to anyone. This particular night, though, he forgot to belch out the smoke trapped in his stomach and returned directly to his entrance post at the restaurant. Harvey pleasantly greeted two couples that came into the restaurant. He gave them a big smile and said, "Good evening. Ah, a table for four. Won't you please come this way?" With each word of his belch-supported voice, puffs of smoke came out of his mouth. Harvey said that he would never forget the startled looks on their faces when he greeted them. As he led them to their requested nonsmoking table, he was amazed that with such a smoky greeting they would follow him anyplace, let alone to a nonsmoking table.

This story took place a little over 50 years ago. Now that smoking has been found to have such a direct relationship to laryngeal cancer, very few laryngectomees today continue to "swallow-smoke" as Harvey did. For those few patients without a voice box who still take in smoke through their mouths and into the stomach, the smoke will remain in the stomach until it is belched out, or, contrary to some rumors of how the smoke finally exits, it will eventually be absorbed through the lining of the intestines.

⌣

Looking Back at Our People with Voice Disorders

Among our eight people with voice disorders, five of them had functional disorders (a seven-year-old girl, two women, and two men); three people had organic disorders (one woman and two men). For the five questions we ask about voice disorders, these eight people with their histories and tales will help us answer each one:

- What are the differences between functional and organic voice disorders?
- Is the pitch of the voice solely dependent on the size of the vocal fold?
- What is meant by vocal hyperfunction?
- Are people with voice disorders generally helped by voice therapy?
- Why are most voice problems not solved by group voice therapy?

I have touched upon most of these questions in the introduction to this chapter and in the beginning of most of the tales. I will add to what we have already talked about, from the perspective of clinical experience and private practice.

Five Questions on Voice Disorders

What are the differences between functional and organic voice disorders?

The stories of our eight patients show clear differences between functional and organic voice disorders. A functional disorder is when a faulty voice is produced by a normal mechanism. Continued faulty use may sometimes lead to physical changes in the larynx; for example, continued yelling and vocal abuse may eventually lead to developing vocal nodules. Penny had her bilateral vocal nodules removed by surgery after months of voice misuse. Such lesions as nodules or polyps are the result of continuous abuse and misuse, and they are considered functional disorders. Both Tom and Coach Fred experienced hoarse voices from continued vocal misuse. Tom spent too much time talking through clenched teeth; Fred developed a near loss of voice from continuous yelling during basketball practice and actual games. Catherine was found to have a normal larynx, but spoke in a higher pitch with baby-sounding resonance. Wanda in her wandering narratives actually spoke most of the time with a near normal-sounding voice. Each of these five people had a functional voice problem with a normal larynx—they needed voice therapy to learn how to use it.

An organic voice disorder is related to some disease or physical change of the larynx. Typical organic changes may include vocal fold paralysis, or lesions of the folds like cysts and papilloma. Thornton experienced major organic changes of his larynx after inhaling an uncontrolled amount of chlorine gas while servicing a swimming pool. His immediate symptom of near-strangulation coughing was followed by permanent tissue changes of his vocal folds. The most serious organic vocal lesions are cancers that involve the lungs, mouth, throat, larynx, or airway. Both Roberta and Harvey experienced extensive cancerous lesions of the larynx, requiring a laryngectomy, or total removal of the larynx. Today, cancer lesions in the airway are often treated with more focal or minor surgery, preceded or followed by radiation therapy. Voice rehabilitation by the SLP usually follows successful medical or surgical treatment of the various physical diseases.

Is the pitch of the voice solely dependent on the size of the vocal folds?

The overall size of the voicing mechanisms (lung capacity, laryngeal size) is the primary determinant of voice pitch range in human development.

After the early cries of the infant and through infancy and childhood, there is a continuous lowering of pitch range as the airway and larynx gradually increase in size. At the time of puberty, there is a dramatic increase of laryngeal size that produces a dramatic lowering of pitch range in both young men and women. The pitch range of the male voice after puberty drops nearly an octave. The female pitch range lowers about half an octave.

The answer to the question is "no." While the overall pitch range is determined by the size of the vocal folds, the changes of pitch when one talks or sings is related to muscular tension changes of the vocal folds. Our lowest note is produced by the vibration of the vocal folds as they contract in length and become the thickest they can become. From this lowest note upward, gradual increases in pitch are produced by gradual stretching and thinning of the vocal folds by other small muscles of the larynx. This gradual progression to higher pitches is the result of this increased thinning, causing a gradual increased tension of the vibrating vocal folds. The highest voice pitch is produced by the vocal folds at their maximum tension and thinness.

What is meant by vocal hyperfunction?

The ENT doctor and the SLP use the term *vocal hyperfunction* to label excessive efforts used by patients when they are using voice. Sometimes it may mean speaking too abruptly or too loudly, or using an inappropriate voice pitch, or there may be excessive coughing and throat clearing. Management and voice therapy for vocal hyperfunction is to "take the work" out of using one's voice.

Seven-year-old Penny was a classic example of vocal hyperfunction and what it can do to sensitive vocal fold tissue. Her parents reported that she was always talking in a loud voice and could often be heard yelling while at play. Eventually, her voice became hoarse most of the time. On a subsequent examination by an ENT, she was found to have bilateral vocal nodules. The nodules were surgically removed (a common practice in the 1960s). However, continued use of loud voice and yelling often produces a recurrence of the nodules. It has been well established that nodules are best treated by the SLP, who uses voice therapy to replace vocal hyperfunction with a normal voice free of excessive effort.

Tom's exaggerated chewing practice with an open mouth was part of his SLP-directed voice therapy program. He had developed voice hoarseness toward the end of his working day as a lawyer. His voice examination found that he did most of his speaking with clenched teeth with very little mouth opening. Voice therapy was successful in helping Tom speak with greater jaw movement and increased mouth opening. His vocal fatigue at the end of his day was eliminated.

Coach Fred's vocal hyperfunction was so severe that his yelling would often cause him to lose his voice after a game. His listeners avoided asking him questions. In our early voice therapy efforts, our counseling to avoid yelling was not successful. The problem was that the coach did not know how to yell without hurting his vocal folds. He responded well to our vocal coaching. We worked on good breath support for saying fewer loud words on one breath. We demonstrated the "barker voice" (increased forward head resonance with a touch of increased nasality), which he now uses whenever he yells.

Are people with voice disorders generally helped by voice therapy?

Both children and adults who experience voice hoarseness without any improvement for more than a week should seek a medical examination by an ENT. The subsequent treatment may be wholly medical or surgical. More often the patient will be referred to an SLP for a voice evaluation and possible voice therapy. The amount of voice therapy is highly individualized, usually depending on the extent and type of voice problem. Our eight people with voice disorders presented some unique problems requiring different therapy approaches by the SLP. Catherine with her high-pitched, "thin" voice got the most out of voice therapy. We saw her twice weekly for six weeks supplemented by daily practice at home. She was able to develop a more posterior focus to her voice, produce a slightly lower voice pitch, and give her voice increased breath support for better loudness. By the end of therapy, she had found the professional voice she had been looking for. She was finally able to interact with her book writers with a voice that sounded like she knew what she was talking about. Tom and Coach Fred were able to end their vocal fatigue by different therapy approaches. Tom never opened his mouth when he spoke. Accordingly, at his first therapy visit we asked Tom jokingly if he had ever been a ventriloquist. We followed up in therapy with extensive mouth-movement exercises and worked on increasing better breath support. Coach Fred felt he needed to yell during basketball practice and even more so in actual games. Unfortunately, the coach did not know how to yell. In voice therapy, he learned to say fewer words on one breath as he talked louder, used an appropriate pitch, and developed a bit more nasality to his voice (this SLP called it the "barker voice"). Fred had a good ear in therapy and was easily able to match our vocal models of the loud barker voice. The coach no longer loses his voice and is able to answer questions after a game with a normal voice.

Penny's story was basically about problems related to asking a voice patient to go on voice rest. After a long prescribed voice rest, some patients, particularly children, have difficulty finding their voices again. It took several weeks before Penny could find her voice again. About two months after surgery, Penny began voice therapy with an SLP in her public school. She experienced good success in developing a normal voice with no return of vocal nodules.

Thornton profited from voice therapy to help his listeners on the phone identify that they were talking to him instead of his wife. Despite a thinning of his vocal folds after inhaling a huge amount of chlorine gas, he was able to lower his pitch a few notes and sound more masculine through therapy tips provided by his SLP.

Both Roberta and Harvey developed functional esophageal voices after their laryngectomy operations. In individual voice therapy, they learned how to direct air into the esophagus, where a vibration in the upper esophagus would produce a sound that they modified as their new substitute voice. Both Roberta and Harvey were able eventually to say six words or more on one extended esophageal vibration. They became active members of esophageal voice support groups, offering great encouragement with their excellent voices to new patients before and after their surgeries.

Wanda provides us a good example of someone who never stops talking. Although she had self-referred herself for a voice evaluation, her persistent need to verbalize made it impossible to do any voice exploration or testing.

Why are most voice problems not solved by group voice therapy?

The SLP frequently works with several people with the same speech problem in small groups. For young children with developmental language problems, group play and interactions with one another are best achieved in group situations. The school SLP working on language and speech problems often places children of similar age and problem into small therapy groups. In hospital and community speech clinics, group therapy often supplements individual therapy for certain speech problems. Over the years, I have grouped together patients with aphasia, motor-speech problems, and stuttering issues.

Group therapy for patients with voice disorders is difficult to achieve for several reasons. We rarely see enough voice patients with the same problem at the same time in one clinical sitting to form a group. Most functional voice problems develop in patients over a period of time, related to different voice abuse-misuse by each particular patient. The uniqueness of the patients' vocal behaviors means they are best treated by individual voice therapy.

In our tales, Tom and Fred with their common histories of vocal hyperfunction could possibly have been grouped with others in a group of men and women with similar voice problems. However, they were seen at different times in different clinics. Thornton with his unique feminine voice problem would not have been a good candidate for grouping with other voice patients. Catherine was an ideal one-on-one patient working closely with her SLP, finding success in producing individual vocal behaviors that gave her a bigger voice. She would not have profited from a group exposure. Wanda would have been a poor group member because of her inability to listen to what anyone else was saying.

Penny, Roberta, and Harvey each profited from group therapy. Penny supplemented her individual voice therapy by joining several other children in a public school voice group. Roberta and Harvey had totally different types of group experiences. More recently, Roberta became an active member of a laryngectomy voice club with its primary purpose to offer support to new patients who had a laryngectomy. Back in Cleveland in the late 1950s, Harvey had been an active member of the Cleveland Lost Chord Club, one of the first laryngectomy support clubs in the nation.

CHAPTER FIVE

~

Tales of Speech Pathology

The stories in this chapter all look at a breakdown of communication. The first four speech pathology stories are about people whose talking differences challenge their listeners to understand them. I then present three tales of difficulty I experienced attempting to get the message out about speech pathology. Next I tell of my visit to evaluate a young man who lost his ability to speak while a prisoner under harsh conditions in a state penitentiary. A breakdown of nonverbal communication is described in our last tale between a hemiplegic airplane pilot and his two frightened passengers.

One of my first post-doctoral clinical jobs was directing a clinical program in stuttering at the Cleveland Hearing and Speech Center. The first two speech pathology tales came out of that experience. "Pith Helmet Therapy" tells briefly of a unique therapy approach with a five-year-old boy who stuttered so badly that he had no functional speech. We then look at the fear of stuttering experienced by a Great Lakes ship captain who describes the power of both negative and positive thinking in "I Can Pa-Pa-Pa-Park a Ship." In the earlier days of the speech pathology profession, it was not uncommon for persons who stuttered to choose speech pathology as their career profession. In "Pick Us Up in the Morning," I describe an unforgettable visit to a graduate program in speech pathology headed by a person who was also a severe stutterer.

In the past thirty years or so, speech-language pathologists have had an increasing role helping transgender (TG) adults find the communication style of their new target genders. We use the term *transgender* for persons who usually over many years were unhappy with their biologic gender, and who now live openly as people confident in their desired gender. In "Victor Now Victoria," we view the successful transition of a male to female TG person.

Playing the role of a speech-language pathologist (SLP) in a medical setting presents many of the challenges and observations we have described in the first four chapters of this book. Beyond a clinical role as an SLP, as one gains more experience within the profession, there are increased opportunities for professional travel, visiting other programs nationally and internationally. Speech pathology is often difficult to explain to people out of the profession. I describe a difficult situation explaining speech therapy to hospital visitors in "Two Minutes, Daniel." SLP speakers (the experts from out of town) often encounter severe auditory and visual limitations from their speaking arenas as experienced in "The L-Shaped Atrium." The unbelievable travel obstacles I experienced attempting to present a voice workshop in Minnesota are recalled in "The Workshop in Duluth." One of the most unforgettable SLP adventures I ever experienced was visiting a patient in a penitentiary. I have for a lifetime wondered what happened to the unfortunate young man with whom I visited in "The State Penitentiary."

A well-known fellow speech-language pathologist and I made a site accreditation visit to a clinical program in Pennsylvania. To get there, we flew to Philadelphia and then spent over an hour and a half in a "stop in every town" airport limousine. After completing the site visit, we asked our hosts if there were a faster way to return to the Philadelphia airport. They suggested that we take a local charter flight. In "Are You the Boys Going to Philly?" we take a fun look back (it was not fun at the time) at the harrowing flight in the Cessna and at the pilot who flew us.

～

Tale 1: Pith Helmet Therapy

Our professional understanding of the problem of stuttering has evolved over time. Normal speech is characterized by a fluent flow of words. Stuttering often begins with a breakdown in this fluent flow, called a dysfluency, with the individual repeating the first sound of a word that he or she is attempting to say. Or the whole word may be repeated at the beginning of an utterance. The repetition may then develop into a prolongation of the first sound of a word, or prolonging the vowel in the middle of the word one wants to say. The dysfluency may evolve further, with the person not able to say the desired sound, often pursing the lips to speak but not able to produce any sound or word. In the speech pathology treatment of stuttering, the open repeating of a whole word is a much better prognosticator for future fluency than the complete blocking of a sound or not being able to initiate a spoken word. The young boy we present here had a complete blocking of his attempts at speech.

Ronnie, age five, was the most severe stutterer I had ever seen. When he tried to talk, he would purse his mouth to say something, but no sound would come out. He was the second child of two severe stutterers who had met in a midwestern university stuttering program. The parents, because of their own lifetime speech struggles, had early concerns about Ronnie's word repetitions, which had started before he was three years old. However, despite their concerns, they waited until he was five before bringing him for a speech evaluation.

At the time of my evaluation, Ronnie could not initiate saying a single word. When I asked him his name, he spent over a minute trying to tell me. Attempting to speak, he would purse his lips, hold his breath, close his eyes, contort his face, and make a few unintelligible grunts. Upon physical examination, we found his voice box (larynx), throat, tongue, and lips to be normal, fully capable of producing normal speech. He was tested and found to have normal hearing. He could follow directions quickly and perform well on nonverbal cognitive tasks, indicating that he had good, if not superior intelligence. His problem in communication was his severe stuttering. He could not speak.

In trying to think of something Ronnie could say without struggle, I thought that perhaps he would be able to repeat nonsense sounds after me. So I conceived the idea of "jungle talk," as if we were repeating the sounds of jungle natives. We each wore a jungle hat or pith helmet to create a speaking environment totally different for Ronnie (a situation I now fondly call "pith helmet therapy"). I told him, "Instead of using real words, we'll pretend we're in a jungle in Africa. We'll meet people who speak a different language than we do. When they speak their different words, like 'wagga porpa' (which I said in a loud voice), we'll say 'wagga porpa' right back to them. You put on a jungle hat, Ronnie," I said, offering him a pith helmet. I then put on a pith helmet, and we looked at each other in a mirror, each wearing our jungle hats, and I said, "You'll be able say jungle talk, Ronnie. You say after what I say."

He looked at me quizzically, as if he wasn't too sure that this was going to work. So I said, "Let's try it. When I speak jungle, you say it back to me." I thought of a pretend jungle word and said, "goggle-babba." Ronnie answered me quickly, "goggle-babba." He looked very surprised and pleased, as this was probably the first utterance in some time that he had been able to say without struggle.

I quickly added more jargon words, and just as quickly he repeated them back to me, showing no facial grimace and no sign of stuttering. After five minutes of his repeating nonsense words after me, Ronnie gave me his own jargon words, asking me to repeat what he said. We spent the rest of the session, modeling nonsense sounds and repeating them after each other.

We wore the pith helmets and did our "jungleeze" repetitions for several therapy sessions. Since what we were saying had no actual form or meaning, Ronnie could willingly repeat it back without any evaluation as to whether he was speaking right or wrong. We used the fluency he experienced in saying the jungle sounds as a means of establishing what normal speech fluency might feel like. I subsequently worked with Ronnie on his stuttering for several years, with good results. As he said years later as a teenager, looking back at our first sessions together, "That time we did that jungle talk wearing those pith helmets was the first time I ever felt happy using my mouth to say anything." Repeating the nonsense jungle words opened up his ability to use his breath and voice in a speech-like manner.

Ronnie is now in late middle age, and most of the time he speaks normally, experiencing only occasional stuttering when in a stressful situation. Most of his listeners do not think of him as having a problem with his speech. In a recent conversation with him about this book, he wanted me to tell this jungle sounds story of when he was a little boy.

～

Tale 2: I Can Pa-Pa-Pa-Park a Ship

Stuttering is generally recognized when an individual repeats a sound as he or she speaks, or prolongs a sound, or gets stuck on a word and seemingly cannot "push" it out. That is the stuttering problem that we hear. A hidden part of the disorder is that most stutterers (the people who stutter) live in extreme fear that they are going to stutter. The anticipation of the stuttering seems to help bring the speech disorder about. Stutterers tell us that they soon "know" when they are going to stutter. They then try to avoid those situations in which the stuttering may occur. Therefore, successful speech therapy for stuttering not only requires modifying the stuttering (repetition, prolongation, or blocking of words), but it also must include counseling that can aid the stutterer in reducing the fear of stuttering and the anticipation of situations where stuttering may occur. Eric, a fifty-year-old stutterer and third-generation Great Lakes ship captain, well illustrates the "knowing I'm going to stutter" aspect of the disorder.

Each year during the winter months, when the Great Lakes were frozen and closed to sea shipping, Eric participated in a weekly adult stuttering group. Eric was a colorful sea captain who liked to tell ship stories, despite his severe stuttering, which at times made his storytelling difficult. Most of the time in the group, however, he would speak normally without stuttering. Suddenly, for reasons that no one could predict, he would stutter, with no word able to come out as he held his breath, tightened his lips, froze his jaw in a fixed position, distorted his face, and closed his eyes. When asked why he would block like that in his speech, he answered, "When certain ideas or topics come up, I know I am going to stutter—and I do."

His remark about knowing he was going to stutter led to a group discussion about anticipation of stuttering, with most group members telling how they try to avoid situations where they know they will stutter. The group agreed that negative thinking will often produce negative results. Fear of stuttering seems to make stuttering happen. The group leader countered that the same thing is true of positive thinking, which often leads to positive outcomes. Knowing and predicting that one will be successful in a task, like putting a golf ball in the cup or selling one's daily quota, seems to be the first step in successfully doing the task.

Eric well illustrated negative and positive anticipation for the group when he said, "When I have to give my na-na-name to someone, I know I'm going to have t-t-t-trouble. And I always stutter. But, hell, take my work for instance. I can stand on the bridge of my 400-foot freighter, which is longer than a football field, and bring her right up to the docking pier. With her lateral thrusters, I know I can park her right within her assigned berth space. I know I can pa-pa-pa-park a ship without trouble. And I do."

Much of the stuttering behavior we see and hear comes about, in part, because the individual knows he or she is going to stutter. This same sureness about a negative outcome seems to help make the negative result occur. If Eric, like other people who stutter, could replace the negative expectation that stuttering will occur with positive thoughts that he will speak fluently, one might predict that he would enjoy more fluent speech. Eric's comment on this last statement: "That's easy for a normal speaker to say."

〜

Tale 3: Pick Us Up in the Morning

Severe stuttering often occurs in particular situations. This is a story of a professional man who stuttered so badly on the telephone that he was often unable to produce a single word, but he talked with near normal fluency in face-to-face communication. Adults with a lifetime of stuttering behind them are often conditioned to anticipate that in a particular speaking situation, they are likely to experience an increase in stuttering symptoms. A particular situation might be when attempting to say one's name, or speaking to an authority figure, or talking on the telephone. The more focal the speaking situation (such as introducing one's self), the greater the possibility of a stuttering occurrence.

Early in the development of speech pathology as a profession, it was not uncommon for a person with a lifetime history of stuttering to become a speech pathologist. Having experienced personal difficulties talking, such men and women made excellent, sensitive clinicians. Some became speech pathologists in the schools, some went into medical settings, and some migrated to university teaching jobs. This particular tale is about a university professor who stuttered and was also the department head of a university audiology and speech pathology training program. The identities of both the university and the department head have been omitted.

In the early 1980s, I served as an accreditation visitor to a number of clinical training programs in speech pathology. Procedures developed by the American Speech-Language-Hearing Association (ASHA) required training programs in speech pathology and audiology to be recertified every few years. To do this, a trio of ASHA members would typically make a site visit to the program, where they would interview both faculty and students, review course offerings, look at clinical records, and draw conclusions relative to the adequacy of clinical supervision. These visitations were long before the instant convenience of email, requiring in those days an intensive postal and telephone exchange in preparation for the visit. The stay usually required two nights: The first night the team reviewed the program's submitted application; the next full day, the trio visited the program on-site, followed that evening by writing their report; early the next morning, the visitors discussed their findings with the department head. The trio of visitors generally left for the airport around noon or early afternoon. The host institution generally made motel/hotel reservations for the three visitors, with each visitor making his or her own travel arrangements.

I was appointed by ASHA to head the site team visiting University X. Each of the three of us arrived at the city airport at different times, with each of us finding our own way to the designated motel near the university. Upon arrival at my motel, I spent some time reviewing the materials this training program had submitted to ASHA. I was most impressed with the thoroughness of the documents. When the other two site team members arrived at the motel, it was my duty to call the program head and arrange for him or someone in his department to pick the three of us up in the morning.

I dialed the home number of Dr. Y. His wife answered, and I said, "This is Dr. Boone, the ASHA visitor to your husband's program. I'd like to speak with John."

"Oh, yes, Doctor Boone, he has been expecting your call. Just a moment."

"OK, thank you," I replied. I waited for 10 or 15 seconds, then heard a noise on the line. I said, "Is this Dr. Y? This is Dan Boone, and our site visitors have all arrived."

"Wun-wun-wun-wun-wun." He repeated this with what sounded like a great struggle, and I realized for the first time that he was stuttering.

I interrupted his repetitions and said, "This is Doctor Boone, and our site team has arrived at the Holiday Inn. We're very impressed with your accreditation application."

"Wun-wun-wun-wun-wun."

I then hoped to get a message to him, beyond our first greeting. "We'd like you to pick us up in the morning at eight o'clock."

"Wun-wun-wun." The tone of his voice sounded a bit more relaxed and seemed to convey agreement.

I wasn't completely sure that he had received my request, so I added, "Will you then, John, pick us up at the Holiday Inn after we've had our breakfast? We'll be at the front door at eight o'clock."

"Aaah, ooo, OK."

It sounded like he got the message, so before hanging up I said, "OK, we'll look forward to seeing you in the morning."

John arrived the next morning in his station wagon at the front door of the Holiday Inn promptly at eight o'clock. In our one-to-one greetings and follow-up conversations, he was most personable and showed only occasional word blocks. Our site visit went very well. His excellent application matched all of our observations. I was impressed with his ability to speak with us all day with relatively normal speech. I confirmed that his severe stuttering was primarily on the telephone when I called him in the evening to talk about the next day's schedule, and I again experienced the same "wun" repetitions.

I have never forgotten this site visit event. I had never realized until that time that there could be such a disparity in fluency between complete blockage on the phone and relatively gifted verbal abilities in "live" conversation.

About ten years later, I had a beer with John at an ASHA convention. He confessed to me his extreme embarrassment in not being able to speak on the phone at the time of our site visit. That episode prompted him to receive successful operant speech therapy. He was eventually able to condition away his expectancy to stutter while talking on the phone. In a recent telephone conversation with him about including his story in this book, he spoke with near normal fluency.

～

Tale 4: Victor Now Victoria

Victor, 35, the son of Russian immigrants, lived the first 18 years of his life in a Bronx housing project. He told this interviewer that he was constantly teased in high school for his feminine behavior and interests, at a time when he felt his inner feelings told him that he was really a female born in a male body. In college, Victor majored in journalism, and upon graduation began a life career as a broadcast journalist, writing for both radio and network television. Finally, at age 30, he elected to become Victoria; she subsequently received continuing hormone therapy and effective electrolysis treatments for arm and facial hair. She then sought our help for feminizing her oral communication.

In her early appointments, we viewed videos of both normal females and TG (male to female) women with whom I had previously worked. Our therapy was based on our observations. We noted that the typical female used far more facial expressions and hand gestures than most males. She was surprised when observing contrasting body postures between men and women, such as adult females crossing their legs while sitting, which is a posture that men do not often do.

Before seeing me for voice therapy, Victoria had tried to elevate her voice pitch to more feminine levels. We actually lowered her pitch down one note from the G3 she had selected to an F3 on the musical scale. Although she was aware that the female voice pitch had to be raised to sound more feminine, she wasn't aware that women use far more pitch changes and intonations in their speech than men do. She then worked successfully to increase her speech inflections by using an auditory playback system where she added pitch and loudness inflections to the short sentences she heard on playback. She also found that her female voice was a bit louder than it should be, so she practiced speaking not only softer but also slower, with a slight breathiness in her voice. She became aware of her tendency to lower her voice pitch at the end of sentences (a typical male voicing pattern), which she found easy to correct by occasionally raising her voice pitch toward the end of a sentence.

It took Victoria no more than six voice therapy sessions (and hours of self-practice) to reach the feminine speech-voice targets that we together had set up as her goal. We then added some minor language changes to the way she spoke. Our overall language change was to use two language patterns common in the speech of most women: (1) use more adverbs and adjectives in her speech; and (2) speak in slightly longer sentences. Perhaps her experience as a professional writer was advantageous for her, as she was able to use feminine language patterns more quickly than the typical male to female TG person.

In the years since we first worked with Victoria, she has adjusted very well to living as an adult female. She elected not to have any genital reconstruction. She developed an active social life by expanding her church activities and serving on the board of a community nonprofit agency. She met another TG woman at the network TV station where she is news director. They began dating and now live together as a couple, owning their own home and several other mutual investments.

Victoria and I have kept in contact since her therapy days. She often volunteers to meet with new male to female transgender women, demonstrating by example her feminine speaking style and continuing career success. She has also joined me at the University of Arizona for several very effective presentations to graduate students studying TG therapies in their voice disorders classes.

〜

Tale 5: Two Minutes, Daniel

As part of my clinical training for a master's degree in speech pathology, I was assigned to Highland View Hospital in Cleveland, Ohio. Highland View in the mid-1950s had two clinical populations: 150 custodial-care patients and about 175 rehabilitation patients, most of whom had chronic neurogenic impairments. As a graduate student, I spent about 18 hours a week there working as a speech pathologist with patients with aphasia or motor speech problems secondary to such neurological diseases as multiple sclerosis, stroke, Parkinson's disease, amyotrophic lateral sclerosis (ALS), or cerebral palsy.

With many of these neurological patients, we worked on improving speech intelligibility and helping some patients to improve swallowing function.

After completing my doctorate, I headed up the speech pathology-audiology program at Highland View. Our section in communication disorders was called Speech Therapy (ST) and was one of four programs (together with Physical Therapy [PT], Occupational Therapy [OT], and Vocational Training [VT]) under the aegis of the Department of Physical Medicine and Rehabilitation (PM&R), headed at that time by a well-known physiatrist, Dr. P.

In the late 1950s, it was important for our profession to maintain its independence from medicine. ASHA wanted the patient referred to the ST program for evaluation and therapy if indicated, with the speech pathologist planning the appropriate treatment. It was different from the physician referrals required for both PT and OT in our PM&R Department. Dr. P. and his assistant physicians would see the patient directly and then prescribe what needed to be done in both PT and OT. Patients with communication disorders were referred by hospital physicians either directly to us, with the prescription usually reading "Speech Evaluation and Therapy, if Indicated," or to our staff audiologist for "Hearing Evaluation."

Dr. P. and I worked out the referral steps very well. With a little explanation and a few examples supplied by me, Dr. P. supported the ASHA position. In time, our Speech Therapy staff included me as director, two full-time speech pathologists (in the 1950s we were not yet called "speech-language pathologists"), and a half-time audiologist.

For the few years I worked there in my first post-doctoral position, I wanted to please the man who had employed me, Dr. P. He also had been most cooperative and helpful working my work schedule around my doctoral classes and helping me to develop a pool of hemiplegic patients for the selection of research subjects. Out of this loyalty, I never complained about the continued stress Dr. P. put me under when he would unexpectedly ask me to demonstrate a patient to hospital staff or to speak to a group of visitors to Highland View.

The PM&R program at Highland View in the 1950s was well recognized nationally and internationally as a prototype program in rehabilitation medicine. Before coming to this country from Poland shortly after World War II, Dr. P. was well known in Europe for his recognized programs in rehabilitation. Consequently, we had many foreign visitors to our program. Usually without any prior warning, Dr. P. would come into our speech waiting room with five or six visitors, or more. Instead of letting me know who they were and where they were from, Dr. P. would typically just say, "Doctor Boone is the head of our speech and hearing clinic."

I would quickly take my cue and give the group a "welcome, please come in."

Dr. P. then might say, "Doctor Boone will now tell you how speech therapy fits in for the patients in the department. You have two minutes, Daniel."

At that particular time in my life, I was able to give a brief but fluent summary about what speech pathology services were all about. If any of our staff were present, I would introduce them. Speech patients were often in the waiting area, and I would introduce them to the visitors as well. All introductions were included in the time block I now fondly refer to as "Two minutes, Daniel."

Dr. P. would stand with the visitors and look at his watch. When the two minutes had expired, Dr. P. would promptly say, "Very well (his frequent statement), and thank you, Daniel," as he escorted the visitors to his next proud site in the PM&R Department.

I look back longingly at those days in the late 1950s at Highland View Hospital in Cleveland, Ohio. Our speech pathologists there had a remarkable impact on improving the lives and communication function of many patients. The positive outcome for many patients that we saw there provided me with clinical insights I have been able to use for a lifetime of speech-language pathology work. And the man who made it all possible for me was Dr. P. I have called him Dr. P. in this brief story because his Polish last name was always difficult for me to spell. I did shed fond tears at his memorial service some 40 years ago.

∼

Tale 6: The L-Shaped Atrium

When one travels out of town to deliver a speech or present a workshop, you play the role of the "out-of-town expert." Over the years, I have presented papers or workshops on such topics as cerebral dominance, therapy scoring, aphasia, voice disorders, and transgender communication. I was often the guest of state associations, therapy groups, and medical organizations, both nationally and internationally. I frequently did not know in advance the room situation in which I would be speaking, how many would be in attendance, what audiovisual equipment would be available, and whether or not I would have amplification. This is a tale of the worst speaking situation that I can remember.

Many years ago, I was invited by the Louisiana Speech and Hearing Association (LSHA) to present a short course at its annual convention, held that particular year in New Orleans. This was many years before PowerPoint presentations. At that time the speaker was required to request a slide projector, screen, a reel-to-reel audiotape recorder, a VHS video playback recorder and monitor(s), laser pointer, and a podium mike/amplifier. I had made the appropriate requests through the LSHA organizer and put my advance efforts into organizing the lecture and the auditory/visual playback presentation.

My particular LSHA presentation was scheduled in the old Sugar Bowl stadium (long before the Louisiana Super Dome was built). I arrived at the massive stadium a half-hour before my presentation was to begin, hopefully to set up the AV equipment and familiarize myself with the room. One of the hostesses led me to where I was to speak. I could not believe the room to which I had been assigned, a large room that could accommodate an audience of several hundred people. The room was L-shaped and tucked outside under the slanting seats of the stadium. It basically had no ceiling but rather an atrium that reached high above us, probably all the way up to the seats in row 40! It appeared to be an acoustic disaster, with the possibility of losing sound up into the atrium.

I soon realized that neither my slides nor my video could be seen by everyone. It was a massive L-shaped room. Even though the podium had been set up at one end of the L, it seemed that more people could hear and see better if the podium were set at the inner angle where the two walls of the L came together. So we had the podium moved to the middle with the seats set in a V-configuration facing each other on each side of the podium. The television monitors and slide screen were moved centrally, which we felt would allow at least 70 percent of the audience to see the visual presentations.

As the LSHA members began to come in and find their seats, we attempted to do a sound check. The microphone was now central in the room at the lower point of the L. The audio speakers faced each other. We immediately experienced the loss of sound floating up to the atrium. There also seemed to be some competing noise coming from the outside hallway.

As I began speaking, much of what I said, even though amplified, seemed to vanish above us. Attempts at increasing loudness produced some reverberation between competing speakers above me on each side of the L-shaped room. People seated within 30 feet of the podium could see and hear without too much difficulty. Beyond that distance from the podium, much of my presentation was lost. Some attendees, who couldn't see or hear the presentation, left the room early. For the presenter (me), it was a nightmare experience that lasted for three hours. For most of the short course, I turned off the amplification and did what I could to project a louder voice. That seemed to improve the sound situation. It took me a day or two to recover my normal voice.

I learned from that frustrating experience in New Orleans the importance of room selection. Lectures in hotel and convention centers are often scheduled in rooms that may compete with the presenters and their auditory and visual presentations. Those of us who host conferences should not be shy in demanding that the presentation setting be workable to both the presenter and the audience. Today, with generations of people raised in a loud, amplified world, audiences have real difficulty listening in less than optimum settings.

~

Tale 7: The Workshop in Duluth

This story could only have happened before the days of smartphones. As frustrating as the speaking circumstances were in "The L-Shaped Atrium," nothing can match the travel difficulties I experienced as a scheduled workshop presenter one February day long ago in Duluth, Minnesota. My home was in Denver at the time, and I had not hesitated to schedule a winter voice workshop in Minnesota. I was used to snow and cold weather during the occasional storms that would come over the mountains of Colorado into Denver. On this particular night, I was scheduled to fly nonstop on Western Airlines from Denver to Minneapolis, but the flight was delayed more than two hours. A severe snowstorm had grounded all Denver aviation for several hours. The flight delay gave me several hours to go over my notes, my slides, and the written summaries of several videos I would be presenting the next afternoon in Duluth. My presentation review in the Denver airport was the last event under my complete control for the next few days.

My plane landed in Minneapolis around one-thirty in the morning. After claiming my luggage, I ventured out to the curb to find some kind of transportation to my airport motel. The digital temperature gauge outside the airport registered 15 degrees below zero. While waiting for a cab, I experienced icicles forming in my nose, blocking the normal passage of air. I literally could blow out small tapered icicles, then breathe normally for a few minutes before the ice again closed my nostrils. I waited about 15 minutes before a cab came and delivered me "half-frozen" to my motel.

In the morning I ventured to the airport rental car lot, as I had planned to drive the approximate 150 miles to Duluth, where I would find the Duluth

School Headquarters Building, the site of my afternoon workshop. The rental car was plugged into a "block heater," and since I had never before used such a heater to keep the engine from freezing after parking, the rental personnel showed me how to plug in the parking lot heater when I reached my destination. The car was equipped with metal stud snow tires, and after reviewing the highway map with the rental staff, they felt that I would have no difficulty driving on the four-lane highway to Duluth.

The highway had been plowed, and there were continuous mounds of the plowed snow stacked, sometimes higher than 15 feet, along the outside lanes. It started to rain, producing an instant layering of ice. To secure better traction, I remembered how we drove in Colorado mountain snows, keeping the car's right wheels pushed against the plowed snow piles, which provided the vehicle needed traction. Every now and then, the car would hit an icy patch, and I would experience some fishtail swirling on the highway. In contrast to my driving struggles, I remember hearing and seeing a northbound passenger train streaking alongside the highway on its uninterrupted rush to Duluth. The ice-snow combination delayed my Duluth arrival about 90 minutes later than I had planned. By consulting my map and asking directions at a gas station or two, I eventually found the Duluth School Headquarters Building.

I found the parking lot on one side of the building. It had stopped raining by then, and a light snow was falling. I could spot the vertical block heaters spaced every two open spaces in the parking lot. I parked the car in the lot, placing the engine heater on top of the engine block. Since my watch told me the workshop was to begin in about 30 minutes, I forgot about finding lunch somewhere. All my workshop materials fit nicely in my Italian leather attaché case, which, stepping around the drifts of snow, I carried to the front door. Posted on the door was this notice: THIS BUILDING IS CLOSED. BECAUSE OF THE ICE STORM, THE BOONE VOICE WORKSHOP HAS BEEN CANCELED.

I realized why the parking lot was nearly empty.

These were the days before computer-generated email and cell phones. There was no way that my hosts could have reached me in Minneapolis. After finding a diner and almost a four-hour wintry drive back to Minneapolis, I reached the airport car rental agency. I had a ten o'clock night flight scheduled back to Denver. To make my disappointing day complete, my return Western Airlines flight to Denver was canceled. I was able to find a room again in the same motel, returning back to Denver the next day.

A few years later, at a benefit luncheon in Denver, I met by accident Robert Six, president of Western Airlines, and I enjoyed telling him briefly about my trip to Duluth and his late and canceled flights. I was more interested, however, in meeting his famous wife, the celebrated Broadway singing star, Ethel Merman.

⌇

Tale 8: The State Penitentiary

Consulting in speech pathology can take the professional SLP to many different settings. One setting that I will always remember was a penitentiary in Kansas in the mid-1960s. I was asked by a neurologist at the University of Kansas Medical Center to evaluate a prison inmate who had just acquired a sudden inability to speak, "possibly an expressive aphasia."

My only referral information was the patient's name (we'll call him Carl) and a brief description of the young man's medical problem. Apparently, while undergoing an examination in the prison hospital for a bladder infection, Carl suddenly lost consciousness. Upon awakening, he had no speech and was tentatively diagnosed as having "expressive aphasia."

It was a short but confusing drive from Kansas City, Kansas, north to the prison. Since there are several prisons clustered in the area, I found it somewhat confusing following the signage to be sure I arrived at the correct prison. Near the prison entrance, I made the mistake of parking my car in a yellow zone not far from the entry gates. As I got out of the car, I heard several cries of "halt," followed by "state your purpose." I then saw on the roof of the two-story entrance building two armed guards pointing their rifles at me. "State your purpose," one of them yelled again.

I yelled back, "I am Dr. Daniel Boone, and I've come to examine a patient in your hospital." (I realized immediately that my historical name might well work against me.)

"You can't park there, Doctor. You'll have to drive over to Special Visitors Parking. We'll have guard escorts there to meet you."

I drove by the front entrance and parked in a small lot marked SPECIAL VISITORS PARKING. As I was getting out of the car, two armed guards approached me, and one of them requested, "Let's see your Special Parking Pass."

"I don't have any special permit, but I have been asked by the warden to examine a prisoner who has lost his speech." Neither guard interrupted me, so I continued, "My name is Doctor (as long as I said 'doctor' I figured they would think I was a legitimate visitor) Boone. I've come to see Carl—in the prison hospital."

Both men answered, "We can't let you in without a special permit, and we cannot let you park here, either." Taking a two-way radio off his hip, one guard said, "Tell me your name again and we'll call it in."

"Daniel Boone. I'm a speech doctor."

After what seemed to be many minutes of waiting and listening to them make fun of my name, the guard told me, "We can issue a 411 that'll cover your car, and Carleton here," pointing to the other guard, "can take you to the main post."

Carleton and I walked to the main gate of the penitentiary, where we were met by several other guards. As the guards accompanied me to the warden's office, we walked through a series of clanging metal gates that would lift upward as we walked under them to the next gate. The whole scene reminded me of an old George Raft movie. I was impressed with how difficult it was to access the warden's office from the inside, thinking how impossible it would be to escape back through the corridors we had just entered.

The prison doctor was waiting for me inside the warden's office along with the warden himself. Both men reviewed Carl's history, with the doctor elaborating, "We examined his bladder by inserting a catheter in his penis. The minute the tube got in there, the boy keeled over in a deep faint. He laid on the floor unconscious with a tube up his cock, completely out of it. When he woke up, he couldn't find his voice. And he hasn't spoken a word in ten days. We want you to see if this is some kind of aphasia or if the guy is giving us a fake reaction."

The doctor and two guards then took me to the prison hospital, which seemed to be in the middle of the prison's central courtyard. Once again I was reminded of a George Raft movie, as I watched more than 20 prisoners breaking rock boulders with picks and sledgehammers, under the close supervision of several guards. As we walked by the prisoners, several of them directed obscenities my way. The doctor explained to me, "They're looking at you as a brand-new queen. This place is divided between kings and queens. The nice guys like doctors, sales guys, or embezzlers are the queens, and tough guys and second-timers are the kings. This Carl guy you're going to see is a decent-mannered kind of guy, which makes him automatically a queen."

Carl appeared to be in his mid-20s, a mild-mannered and cooperative man who had been sentenced to prison on an embezzlement conviction. In just a few minutes, I was aware that he understood everything that was said to him. Unlike the responses of a typical patient with aphasia, my subsequent testing found that he could read silently, write, and follow spoken instructions with quick, normal ability. His attempts at using voice and talking, however, met with total failure. He was even unable to count aloud in a rapid series, which many aphasic patients are able to do. When asked to repeat "ah" after me, he could only posture his mouth with no voice. It became apparent to me that Carl did not have aphasia, but symptoms of conversion aphonia. What he needed was a brief exposure to voice therapy with strong psychological support and counseling.

Following my 40-minute examination, I was escorted with the doctor back to the warden's office. As I entered his office, before I could say anything or write my evaluation, the warden asked me, "Does he have aphasia?"

"No, I don't think so," I replied.

Before I could say anything else, the prison doctor interrupted, "It's just what I told you, Warden, there's some kind of hysteria going on here. This guy doesn't have aphasia any more than you do, sir."

The warden's response to my quick answer will always haunt me. He concluded our evaluation by saying, "Well, we'll get that boy to talk. Thank you, Doctor, for confirming what we pretty well knew." Turning to his lieutenant, the warden ordered, "I want that Carl guy out of the hospital and put on work detail, words or no words."

I have long wondered whatever happened to Carl after my useless visit. I know that if I had not been trapped into saying a quick "no" to the question, "Does he have aphasia?" I could have made a favorable case for Carl. I would have liked to tell the warden that many people react to extremes of stress by being unable to speak. Such mutism is not willful or done with deliberation. It is usually a temporary condition of speechlessness that responds well to counseling and psychological support. I wish that I had been able to offer that to Carl.

⁓

Tale 9: Are You the Boys Going to Philly?

It is difficult to put into words the flight travel I experienced on an ASHA clinical certification visit to a hospital setting some 40 miles west of Philadelphia. A particular body in ASHA, the Professional Services Board (PSB) at the time, asked me and another professional man (Dr. M) to make a visit to a clinical program that had requested PSB renewal certification. To get to the site, I flew from Tucson to Philadelphia, and then took a 90-minute van ride on a shuttle to the visitation city. My visitation colleague, Dr. M, had a later but similar 90-minute shuttle ride from Philadelphia to our visitation city.

On the night before our clinic visit, as we were reviewing the submitted program materials, we both agreed that our 90-minute shuttle ride, stopping seemingly at every small town, should be avoided on our return to Philadelphia, if at all possible. After voicing our shuttle complaint to the staff of the speech and hearing clinic, they quickly identified for us a much faster way to return to the Philadelphia airport. There were five or six pilots in town; they collectively owned their own Cessna, and they took turns on particular days to serve as an air taxi service, taking up to three people wherever they needed to go. Our host director called the air service and arranged for both Dr. M and me to fly back to Philadelphia early the next afternoon.

After lunch with our program host the next day, she drove us to the city airport, leaving us with our luggage at a small one-room "terminal." As Dr. M and I waited by the empty building, we became concerned about a possible breakdown in our planned travel. Finally, a large black Chrysler drove up beside us and parked in the adjacent parking area. An older man, probably in his 60s, got out of the car with some difficulty, and we quickly identified that he had a left-sided hemiplegia. His left arm appeared paralyzed, and he walked with what looked like a partially paralyzed left leg, with his foot held up at a right angle by a short leg brace.

He walked with a severe limp toward us and asked, "Are you the boys going to Philly?" We nodded and attempted to introduce ourselves, but he picked up our two cloth pieces of luggage and said, "Follow me to that brown and white Cessna parked over there." We followed him, figuring that he hung around the airport collecting monies from passengers, or doing some airport maintenance work, or despite his left-sided paralysis of arm and leg assisted passengers with their luggage.

He opened the right door of the four-seat Cessna, struggled to put our luggage in the storage space behind the two rear seats, and then laughingly added, "We need to put your carry-on cases back with your luggage. We won't have any time for you to do any office work before you get to Philly."

We each had an attaché case, which we handed to the airport stranger, who placed them back with our luggage. As we stood beside the Cessna, both of us began to feel a bit apprehensive, but particularly Dr. M, who had a strong fear of flying.

The airport handyman turned out to be our pilot. He directed Dr. M to sit in the right rear seat and said to me, "I'm going to ask you to fly captain's left chair today. You get up and slide across to the left chair. I'll follow you up and fly right chair."

Both Dr. M and I followed his directions without challenge. Not until we were belted in our respective seats and the pilot had closed the right door with his normal right hand did we each appreciate the possible seriousness of our situation. As the pilot slid the right air-vent window open, he said to me, "Loosen that window clip beside you and slide her open. We need a little fresh air in here."

He was obviously aware of our apprehensions, and before switching on the engine, he gave us some explanation. "You see, I am having trouble moving my left arm. It all started three months ago when I was a victim of a head injury from a total equipment failure. I'll be getting my renewal physical in a couple of months. You have no worry about me flying you to Philly, as I've been flying these birds for over 40 years. I'm known in these parts as Captain Bill. The hardest thing I've had to deal with since the crash is getting my feet to work the pedals. You probably know that flying an airplane is all footwork. My left leg now works everything down there fine. My left arm just sits on the yolk, but I pull her back or push her down with my right arm. So there's no problem moving the yolk." I could not believe the nightmare Captain Bill was telling us.

"As I told you, I go up for my physical renewal in a couple of months, and in the meantime, I've learned to fly again like any normal guy. They told me you were a couple of speech doctors, and as you hear me talk, I'm sure you'd say I'm a normal talker? We have to be normal talkers, working the radio and all."

I am sure that Dr. M was thinking along with me, "The guy has had head trauma, talks free of dysarthria, doesn't seem to have aphasia or trouble with words, but what about his cognition? Has he lost any of his mechanical abilities or practical intelligence?" Our private thoughts were interrupted as Captain Bill started the engine.

We immediately began taxiing on the grass beside the paved runway. I thought this was in error and said, "It looks like we're taxiing on the grass. Shouldn't we be moving over on the pavement?"

"No, we never taxi on a runway. We stay on the grass till we reach the end of the runway. We wouldn't want to interfere with incoming traffic landing down on the runway." It was comforting to me to hear his logical explanation.

Captain Bill then explained to me why he had me sit in the left chair, which is usually the chair that the pilot occupies. "I asked you, Doctor, to sit in the captain's chair so you could help me with my left arm. When I taxi to the end of the runway, I'd appreciate it if you'd lift my arm up to the yolk so my hand can grab the yolk at the same height as my right hand. When we get enough air speed, I'll pull back on the yolk and we'll lift off the ground.

When I tell you to 'pull her down,' I'll want you to remove my hand from the yolk and let my arm fall down on my lap. It's most important that you don't touch the yolk, so remember to keep your hand off the yolk, and just release my hand from the yolk so I can lower my arm down." He repeated the instruction in a loud voice. "When I yell 'UP,' lift my left arm up to the yolk. When I yell 'DOWN,' pull her down. That's why you're flying left chair, Doctor. Help me with the dead arm." He then asked me to practice the lifting up and the down maneuvers a few times, after which he commented, "Good moves, Doctor, just perfect."

I could not believe what Captain Bill was asking me to do. At that point, I believed our "survival" depended on my arm assistance, so I yelled back my confirmation for lifting or lowering his left arm. As he taxied to the end of the runway, he yelled further instructions to both of us: "Once we're airborne, both of you look to the right and to the left, up and down, for other air traffic. Let me know what you see!"

At the end of the runway, he revved up his engine for a few minutes. Finally, he yelled to me as he released the brakes, "Lift her up!" I lifted his arm to the yolk, and we began increasing our speed down the runway. We were soon airborne, and I followed his instruction to lower his arm from the yolk. I was relieved when he pulled back on the yolk with his right arm, and we seemed to have experienced a normal takeoff. I could hear a very nervous Dr. M in the rear seat let out some low-voice approval.

As we gained altitude, Captain Bill continually acknowledged both Dr. M's and my warnings about sighting distant aircraft, usually saying, "I see him, boys, thanks for the look." The actual flight seemed to be quite routine. I felt that Captain Bill worked the radio and Philadelphia tower instructions with normal procedures, acknowledging the controller's instructions and following them promptly.

As we started our descent into the big Philadelphia airport, Captain Bill was wearing his headphones and spoke in a louder voice to us, "Watch for the big commercial jets that we don't get in their way. I see a big American jumbo coming beside us. They have their own runways and we have our own small one. If you see any of them crossing into our landing space, let me know!"

Just before we touched down, Bill asked me to "lift her up," and I promptly raised his left arm and hand to the yolk. We landed without any problems, eventually taxiing off to a tarmac used for parking small planes.

As Bill opened the right door and climbed down, stepping onto the wing, he said to us, "Now, that wasn't so bad, was it? It sure as hell must have beat riding all day in that shuttle van they use." He helped me out first and then helped Dr. M step down to the ground. I still remember how good it felt to be standing on the ground again.

As he took our bags down from the plane, he said, "Thanks for flying with us today. The lady at the hospital has already paid for you." Raising his right arm and pointing, he said, "You doctors just follow the arrows and you'll get to the main Philly terminal. I'm going to say goodbye to you now 'cause I got to get going back to where we came from." We each said thanks and shook his right hand, and he added, "I'll miss you helping me with my left arm, Doctor. Whenever I got anyone flying with me since the accident, I always appreciate some extra help to keep things steady."

Neither Dr. M nor I will ever forget our Cessna flight to Philly. The last time I saw Dr. M at a speech-language pathology convention in Chicago, I asked him with a straight face, "Do you ever hear from Captain Bill?"

⌢

Looking Back at Our People with Speech Pathology Problems

It was difficult for me to select five questions that can be answered by looking back both at our patients' stories and at the complex field of speech-language pathology. The questions are:

- Can stuttering begin at the preschool level?
- Does fear of stuttering keep the problem alive in people who stutter?
- What are some of the communication changes transgender people must make in their change from biologic gender to their preferred gender?
- What is the impact of emotions on the voice?
- How do communication defects affect our use of language

In this chapter we have had a wide age range of people in our tales, from young Ronnie, age five, to Captain Bill, probably in his mid-60s. Our first question looks at one commonly held view on how stuttering gets started in a child.

Five Questions on Speech Pathology

Can stuttering begin at the preschool level?

Ronnie's parents told us in his evaluation workup that he began to show what sounded like stuttering before he was three years old. Since both parents had a history of stuttering, they were aware that sometimes stuttering ran in families. However, normal children at this age show some struggle as they are developing their language and speech. They begin combining the names of things (nouns) with action words (verbs). In their play, their words are put together well. Sometimes when they are talking to adults, though, their words may be said with some struggle. According to some SLPs, how adults react to the child's early word struggles is sometimes the genesis of a later stuttering problem. Other children seem to develop stuttering from a persistent problem in expressing their thoughts into fluent speech. Ronnie at age five had already stuttered for a few years, and he had already learned to expect struggling for everything he wanted to say.

In both private and group speech therapy, Eric had memories of stuttering for a lifetime, beginning before he even started school. He developed a continuing awareness of the places and situations where he was going to stutter. If he couldn't avoid the situation, he told me something like, "I'd just go ahead and plow through them trying to talk." In several talks with our SLP friend, John, he remembered missing kindergarten because his mother thought other children would tease him badly because of his stuttering. He thought that his personal success in overcoming his stuttering problem in speech therapy over the years was the primary factor motivating him to become a speech-language pathologist. Dr. John not only treated many people who stuttered over the years, but at the university level he taught courses and did research in stuttering. He believes there are multiple causes of stuttering, which means there is no one effective treatment for all stutterers. Similar to his own stuttering experience, he felt that for most stutterers, the problem of stuttering first shows itself during the preschool years.

Does fear of stuttering keep the problem alive in people who stutter?

People who stutter tell us that the act of stuttering is a most unpleasant event. The typical listener does not know how to react to the stuttering—he or she may look the other way, or may try to provide the struggled word, or may offer advice to slow down or take a big breath. The stutterer has a natural need to avoid these reactions. He soon learns to fear certain words or situations where he *knows* he is going to stutter. This is why most effective speech therapy for stuttering is twofold: (1) modify the stuttering act itself; and (2) work to minimize avoidance and fear.

Ronnie's speech fear was saying anything. He could use his mouth well for everything but talking, such as chewing and swallowing food. I can well imagine the fear he must have had being brought to a speech clinic to show people how he stuttered. When asked to play talk in "jungleeze," he had no previous fears for such mouth noises. He spoke the nonsense words freely. We were able to establish some actual language melody, or prosody, by his forward saying of nonsense words. After a few sessions using nonsense words, we were able to bridge over to more conventional therapy.

Over many years, Captain Eric developed awareness of words and situations where he would experience difficulty speaking. Anticipating the word struggles ahead, he had become a master of substituting words for the ones he knew he would stutter (called *circumlocution* by SLP professionals). In speech therapy, he learned a few methods for controlling his stuttering blocks so that he could "go ahead and stutter" in such an easy way that it didn't interfere with his communication with other people. Captain Eric was a strong group member in expressing his belief that his fear of stuttering was part of the reason he still stuttered.

Professor John talked about a lifetime of stuttering. He had become a fluent speaker by following therapy techniques and by overcoming his fear of stuttering in various situations. When I first met him during a professional visit to his university program, he seemed to have but one fear situation remaining: talking on the telephone. He had been conditioned over time to expect difficulties talking to someone on the phone. Since that visit, he has been able, through operant conditioning, to eradicate his fear of the telephone. In a recent phone conversation with John, I heard normal speech fluency.

What are some of the communication changes transgender people must make in their change from biologic gender to their preferred gender?

A change of pitch level is only one of the changes a transgender (TG) person must do in making the gender switch in communication. Among normal adults, women have higher-pitched voices (a little more than a half-octave) than men the same age. For example, at age 40 the typical woman's habitual voice pitch is around G3 on the musical scale (200 Hz); the habitual pitch of men the same age is near A2 (110 Hz). In our transgender tale, Victoria, in her attempt to sound more feminine, first came to see me with a voice pitch several notes higher than women her age. It turned out the best voice for her was just two or three notes higher than her previous masculine voice.

Changing pitch level for those making female to male voice changes is much simpler than when we work with the male to female voice. The female voice can be dramatically lowered by hormonal therapy (primarily testosterone) with additional speech therapy suggestions. Hormonal therapy (primarily estrogen) for the male to female voice has no pitch-rising effects. In my work with TG persons, I put less emphasis on pitch change and more attention to other factors for females: increasing facial expression and gesture, more descriptive words, increased speech rate, elevating pitch toward the end of sentences, and increasing the use of pitch inflections for females.

For my female to male TG people, I attempt to move them in the opposite direction of those factors just listed for increasing femininity.

An important part of changing communication style in the TG population is for the new TG person to get to know other successful TG people. Victoria was so comfortable and successful with her feminine communicating style that she became one of my favorite visitors to meet new male to female people. She also met with university graduate students, who were impressed not only by her speaking ability, but also by her career and personal life successes.

What is the impact of emotions on the voice?
While the larynx has a steady primary role of protecting the airway, its role in providing phonation is much more vulnerable. Its protective role in humans is similar to all other vertebral animals—protecting the airway on inhalation. Compared to the subtlety of human phonation, animal phonations are grossly similar in duration and sound similarly across the species. For humans, shadings in the voice can show the emotional or psychological state of the person. People who are anxious or under stress can often hide the condition every way but vocally. Such emotions as fear or anger or even happiness can be heard in the human voice.

Emotionality seems to trigger changes in the overall physiology of voice production. There appear to be slight changes in airflow through the larynx shaped by changes in muscle tension within the larynx and tension changes in the resonating structures above the vocal folds. In its mild form, a person may have a normal voice most of the time, but when an unexpected event happens, he or she may produce an audible change of voice or possibly experience a complete loss of voice. We have all witnessed the impact of someone not being able to speak after hearing about a close relative's death, or someone losing his voice on hearing the good news of winning the lottery. On television, we frequently see the winner on an award show unable to find his or her voice in response to questions.

Sometimes the poor voice continues, and the SLP calls it *functional dysphonia*. Upon physical examination, both respiration and the larynx are normal. Similar to some of the voice patients we read about in chapter 4, most patients with functional dysphonia do very well recovering their voices in voice therapy. The total absence of voice experienced by someone with a normal larynx is labeled as *functional aphonia*. Their treatment with an SLP is usually brief, with the patients making an excellent recovery of normal voice.

Carl, the young man who lost his voice from the medical trauma in the penitentiary, is an example of a psychiatric disorder, *conversion aphonia*. This sudden loss of voice, despite having a normal larynx, seems to originate when the patient experiences a sudden intolerable emotional or physical event. This is an extreme example of the vulnerability of the human voice to the impact of emotions. In conversion aphonia, the patient may lose consciousness and awaken unable to speak or use voice. No matter how he or she tries, they cannot find voice. Fortunately, it has an excellent prognosis when treated by an SLP. The literature tells us that the sooner it is treated, the better the prognosis; the protective nature of the lack of voice must be interrupted. Treatment for conversion aphonia by the SLP parallels the treatment used in functional aphonia. Unfortunately, for young Carl no treatment was available.

How do communication defects affect our use of language?

In the four previous chapters of this book, we have looked at people with many different defects in communication. We have looked at such problems as word-finding searching, speech and voice defects, and talking rhythm problems that may interfere with communication. Not only do listeners have difficulty understanding what the speaker with a communication defect is trying to say, but the speaker, because of hearing loss, aphasia, or dementia, also may not fully understand what is being said back to him. As we look back in this chapter, for example, we can appreciate how the problem of stuttering seriously impaired the use of expressive language by the three people who stuttered. Our transgender woman, Victoria, needed to use the language and communicative style that promoted her femininity to her listeners. Captain Bill with his left hemiplegia used his language skills to compensate for his lost motor skills required for flying an airplane.

Our use of spoken language works in two ways: We speak, and we listen. In this book, we presented the talking and listening problems of older people with either aphasia or dementia. The problem of communication breakdown is shared by the listeners who are trying to understand what our patients are trying to say. Communication difficulties like a speech defect (such as dysarthria) or a voice problem (such as dysphonia) increase the difficulty for listeners trying to understand what is being said.

While speaking and understanding what is being said are what oral language is all about, graphic language (reading and writing) is perhaps the more stable of the two language systems. Happenings of the past and present can be remembered in our written language. This author offers this simplified definition of language: oral, graphic, and gestural symbols used by a common group that represents actions, feelings, and things of the past, present, and future. Probably all of our patients in our tales have memories of the past, including the people with dementia. Part of the way we retrieve memories from the past is through the recall of language memories. Our abilities to think abstractly and plan for the future are possible by the use of language thinking beyond the present. This ability for using language to look at the future and to plot future happenings appears to be a unique human ability in contrast to the other animal species of the world.[1]

It is use of oral language in the present that is most reduced by communication disorders. While the impaired speaker may have problems expressing his thoughts, his listener may also have real difficulty understanding what he is trying to say. The effective use of language between speaker and listener is often compromised by the communication defect.

~

CHAPTER SIX

Management of Communication Disorders

Looking back at the many tales in the previous chapters, there is a diversity of patients with a wide variety of communication disorders. With the exception of two patients (Bonnie and Ronnie), all the other people in the tales were adults (18 and older) seen by speech-language pathologists (SLPs) in either medical or university clinics. None of our patients were seen primarily for a hearing loss by audiologists, which is why there are no tales about people with hearing loss in this book.

For the reader, we need to validate who is a speech-language pathologist. In health-related communication disorder clinics, the SLP plays a primary role. In this chapter, management suggestions and discussion will be limited to the type and kind of patients presented in our many tales. All of these stories were told by SLPs. The American Speech-Language-Hearing Association (ASHA) designates the terms *health care* and *college-university care* to categorize about 45 percent of certified SLPs working with adult communication disorders of speech, language, and voice. Most of our patients were seen in such health-related settings as nonresidential, hospital, or residential. A few people were outpatients in university speech clinics.

Finding a Speech-Language Pathologist (SLP)

According to ASHA in 2017, among its 191,000-plus members, 52 percent of them are certified SLPs working with children in early intervention, preschool, and school age (K-12). The academic and professional requirements for SLPs who work in the schools are the same as for those who elect to work in health care: two years of intensive graduate study in an ASHA-approved program, passing comprehensive departmental exams, and passing an ASHA-sponsored clinical exam (praxis). At this point, the successful graduate selects a school or medical setting for his or her clinical fellowship year (minimum of 36 weeks). After completing the clinical fellowship, the new SLP becomes eligible to apply for ASHA's clinical certification; after receiving this certification, the SLP will use this signature display: "Jane Doe, CCC-SLP." The selection of job setting is highly individualized. Fortunately, for the new graduate there appears over the years to always be a need for more SLPs in both school and medical settings.

Most states in the United States require state licensing for the SLP. Some states may also require a special certificate to work in particular settings, such as in the public schools. In the medical setting, the SLP works closely with other medical professionals, such as physicians (neurologists, otolaryngologists, plastic surgeons, orthopedic surgeons) and other medical rehab specialists (physical therapists, occupational therapists, social workers, etc.). For families and friends of people with communication disorders, the list of possible helpful professionals can be overwhelming. However, for problems talking, the SLP is probably the best-trained professional among other health care professionals to offer advice on appropriate professional care.

There continues to be confusion among patients (particularly among older patients) and their families about the title of speech-language pathologist. Up until the late 1960s, we were called *speech therapists* or *speech clinicians*. In the 1970s, the official name was changed to *speech pathologist*. By 1980, ASHA governing bodies changed the official name to *speech-language pathologist*, which is our professional name today. There has also been an official change by insurance companies and government agencies for the name of therapy that the SLP provides, from *speech therapy* to *speech-language services*. This therapy name change came about because both PT (physical therapy) and OT (occupational therapy) treatments are prescribed by physicians. The SLP, by virtue of being the only professional trained in speech remediation, makes his or her own treatment plans. The SLP receives a referral for evaluation directly from the physician. After the examination, the SLP makes the decision for the amount and type of service. Or the patient with a communication disorder may contact the SLP directly, who will then determine if a medical evaluation is needed.

Rehabilitation for Communication Disorders

Before presenting some discussion and steps for adult rehabilitation of selected communication disorders, the reader might re-read the few preceding paragraphs that describe the academic and professional training of the SLP. He or she is the most qualified professional to offer advice and counsel about problems of speech, language, and voice.

Faulty advice can come from many sources, whether it was asked for or given freely without request. For example, family and patients may actively seek advice from the local church choir director or from a teacher of singing. Or recognizing the superior speaking ability of local clergy, they might ask the family minister for advice about a talking problem. Family doctors or dentists often are asked for their advice about an oral communication problem for which they have had only minimal professional exposure.

I have found over time that the most inappropriate advice may come from family and friends. Each person has one's own private talking history, out of which he or she has some personal knowledge about talking. Although this personal talking advice may be helpful for the patient, it can sometimes be harmful, and may delay the patient from seeing a needed professional person, such as an SLP.

Another increasing problem possibly delaying effective treatment are social media, newspaper, and radio-TV commercials. Often, one experiences a series of back-to-back, successive commercials touting cures for endless ailments. Accordingly, physicians report they are bombarded by patients requesting various medical or physical treatments that the patients keep hearing about on television. Fortunately, there are few quick fixes or pills advertised to help someone with a problem communicating.

In a quick computer search, one can find a number of apps available that may focus on aspects of speech and voice. There are continually additions and deletions on app menus, which make it impossible for a book like this to make a specific app recommendation. Family and friends should *not* directly access a speech-voice app, as it may be inappropriate. Rather, follow the advice of an SLP for using specific apps for therapy practice and for improving overall communication skills.

In *Trouble Talking: The Realities of Communication, Language, and Speech Disorders*, a quick look was given to a number of people with communication disorders. This was followed by a few questions related to the disorder, with the answers provided in part by the individuals described in each of the stories told in that particular section. Although glimpses were given of what SLPs do for each disorder (its management or therapy), no direct advice was given. Instead, the reader of this book is given some general advice that could be followed by initiating management and therapy for someone with a communication disorder.

The priority advice is to consult when possible with a speech-language pathologist (SLP). By contacting an SLP in the schools, in a local hospital, or in private practice, the patient or family should be able to find an SLP with the needed clinical experience. Fortunately, there are a number of associations and societies available across the country that can help identify appropriate SLPs and treatment agencies. These agencies are listed alphabetically by name and what they can offer in the "Resources" chapter in this book.

All SLPs are certified members of the American Speech-Language-Hearing Association (ASHA). Besides their professional publications, ASHA has a number of pamphlets and brochures about various communication problems. ASHA has recently developed a new service for the lay public in search of an audiologist or SLP known as ASHA ProFind. Not only will ASHA ProFind help a patient find an SLP in his or her community, but it also answers a number of relevant questions, such as to how to prepare in advance for an audiologist or SLP appointment.

For patients and families who wish to find available local speech and hearing services, telephone directories may list the official name of their state's speech and hearing organizations. State organizations are patterned closely after ASHA. The name listing is usually the name of the state followed by Speech-Language-Hearing Association. In my state, our organization is called the "Arizona Speech-Language-Hearing Association."

In subsequent pages in this chapter, various disorders are briefly presented with practical management steps. Also, family and patients with communication problems related to a specific disorder or disease might wish to Google the name of the disorder and find if there is a friendly association or society to contact. For example, for someone with multiple sclerosis, the National Multiple Sclerosis Society might be helpful. Again, the "Resources" chapter lists national organizations with some description of available resources. Under each organization listed, we have provided the postal address, land phone number, and web page, if available.

Each of the previous five chapters in this book looked at patients with communication problems related to different disorders: aphasia, dementia, neurogenic disorders, voice disorders, and speech pathologies. Here, management strategies for patients and families are presented separately for each of the clinical areas.

Aphasia

Aphasia is caused either by vascular accident (stroke) or traumatic injury to the brain. As presented in chapter 1, the aphasia symptoms are usually the result of damage to the left cerebral hemisphere, often accompanied by right-sided weakness of the right arm and leg. Three of the patients in our tales had rapid spontaneous recovery from aphasia because they received prompt medical attention after experiencing their accident or injury: the nurse Helen, the apple critic Dan, and the group piano player, Keith. Each of these three people recognized the early warning signs that they were having a stroke and were able to receive prompt (within two hours of onset) medical treatment.

A stroke is a sudden interference of blood supply to the brain (cerebral vascular accident [CVA]). The two types of CVA, or stroke, include blockage of blood (ischemia) and hemorrhage. There is also what is known as a "mini-stroke," or transient ischemic attack (TIA). All of our people with aphasia in our tales (except Louie, who had a gunshot injury) experienced sudden language problems from a CVA-caused lack of blood supply to parts of the left cerebral hemisphere.

The sudden and early warning signs of a CVA (WebMD) should signal the need for immediate medical treatment. The sooner the CVA patient receives treatment, the less chance of damage to the brain producing permanent disability. There are five sudden major warning signs (WebMD) of a stroke: (1) unilateral weakness or numbness of face, arm-hand, and leg; (2) confusion or trouble understanding the speech of others; (3) difficulty speaking; (4) changes of vision; (5) severe dizziness. With early and successful medical treatment, the symptoms of aphasia begin to lessen within a few days. Although a complete spontaneous recovery may seem apparent after two weeks, some patients (like Helen in chapter 1) report that sometimes under stress they may still experience a problem of word retrieval.

Aphasia treatment should begin as early as possible after onset.[1] Today, in most hospitals a neurologist and SLP are available to evaluate and begin treatment for the new patient with aphasia. The first obstacles to a planned recovery, however, may be imposed by medical insurance and Medicare. Unlike many of our aphasia patients visited in chapter 1, who received all the speech therapy they needed, aphasia patients today may face serious inpatient and outpatient financial limitations. Fortunately, the hospital SLP can usually make arrangements for individual therapy and eventually for group therapy, meeting perhaps weekly with other people with aphasia.

While there are several professional aphasia organizations that are focused on aphasia research and clinical service, there is one group, the National Aphasia Association (NAA) that advocates for persons with aphasia and their families. Founded in 1987, a focus of the NAA is to help new patients receive the rehabilitation services they need within their home communities. The standards for appropriate aphasia therapy by the SLP are set by ASHA's clinical standards for evidence-based practice (EBP). Aphasia therapy guided by EBP standards includes the integration of the SLP's clinical expertise, patient values, and the best research evidence available for the decision-making process.

Billing procedures for both individual and group therapy for aphasia by Medicaid and Medicare is under the label *speech pathology services*. The initial referral for these services can come from the family physician, a physiatrist, a neurologist, or directly from the SLP.

After initial testing and getting acquainted with the patient and family, individual therapy is planned. Many articles and books have been written on the kind of speech/language therapy that can be offered, depending in part on the type of aphasia presented by the patient. A Google search of books on aphasia therapy and practice workbooks can be overwhelming; the family literature search is probably best directed by the SLP and other rehab specialists, such as the physiatrist. Similarly, the search at the apps store for useful self-practice aphasia-recovery programs is best delayed until it can be directed by the SLP. For aphasic patients who are comfortable with computers, the SLP can assign many apps for both oral and graphic language self-practice.

Each of the 12 people in chapter 1, "Tales of Aphasia," received traditional individual and group aphasia therapy. Emphasis was given to finding residual language functions and exploiting them in "can-do" therapy. Patients were asked to use maximally what they could still say. Auditory feedback was used heavily, from close auditory feedback to listening to and singing the lyrics of popular songs from one's younger years. Some innovative and effective modifications in recent years, added to traditional language retraining, have been achieved by integrating more nonlinguistic therapies.[2] It appears that some return of language function can be facilitated by attention given to nonverbal short-term and long-term memory, emotions, executive function, and nonverbal visual processing. These nonlinguistic processes coupled with spoken language tasks in aphasia therapy are well illustrated in the Cahana-Amitay and Albert book.

In our story of an unusual but effective aphasia group session, "Honolulu Annie," we uncovered a number of spontaneous interaction patterns between the six members of the group. Bill and Joe reacted to Annie's wheelchair dancing with their same perseverative responses, but spoken with very happy inflection patterns. The other three people in the group made comments using the words they were able to say as Annie sang her nonsense-sounding Hawaiian words. This particular scene was fostered by the SLP to encourage social interaction between group members. While social interaction is an important part of aphasia group therapy, conversational practice is equally important. The SLP is aware of each patient's linguistic ability and offers the patient, through prompting and actual situations, a platform to say what he or she is able to say. The typical person with aphasia quickly becomes accustomed to feeling misunderstood. Speaking success in the group is a welcomed relief.

If enough other people with aphasia were around, our new patient would be scheduled with other aphasic patients in a group setting. Ongoing individual therapy is supplemented by ongoing group therapy. After completing individual therapy, ideally the patient would be able to join others in a group situation (hopefully at least weekly). The group setting allows the patient to see how other group members are doing and gives the patient the opportunity to speak with understanding listeners. And the existing group plays an important role for the new patient with aphasia.

Before we leave the topic of aphasia and left hemisphere lesions, we must remember briefly our left hemiplegic Cessna pilot, Captain Bill. He did not have aphasia. His right brain damage came from accident trauma, which produced his left-sided paralysis of arm and leg. Bill did show a few of the psychological symptoms often attributed to right hemisphere dysfunction, such as denial of disability with an exaggerated self-centeredness. At least he was a great help flying us back to Philadelphia.

Dementia

There were two patients, Dr. Sam and Pearl, in chapter 2, "Tales of Dementia," who well illustrate the progressive ravages of dementia. Even as a college professor, Dr. Sam was able for several months to hide his increasing confusions and memory loss caused by Alzheimer's disease by keeping detailed calendars and writing notes to himself. In time, his behavioral confusions began to be visible to others. This is the typical course of Alzheimer's. In time, the patient becomes less aware of his limitations, and the concern transfers over to the family. A similar progression of symptoms was experienced by Pearl, whose battle with vascular, or multi-infarct, dementia began when she experienced difficulties dressing herself. She soon required dressing help from her spouse plus increasing help in overall self-care and in most of her attempts at housekeeping. As her confusions increased, she lost the ability to initiate any responsible behaviors, requiring several years of supervision in a memory care facility before her death.

The SLP can be of assistance to the family in two ways: (1) evaluate the patient's memory and language function as part of a medical/psychological diagnostic evaluation; and (2) in early stages, develop and provide verbal and nonverbal memory materials and speech practice. In suspected or early developing dementia, the SLP should first determine the patient's auditory acuity and visual abilities. It has been observed in older patients that severe hearing loss can sometimes be the cause of confusion. With proper hearing amplification, the patient is no longer confused. After checking the patient's hearing and vision, the SLP evaluates oral function for chewing/swallowing and then administers a few relevant speech/language tests developed for identifying dementia.[3]

There appears to be no definitive medication or behavioral therapy that can reverse the course of dementia.[4] Fortunately, there are things that can be done to slow down the advance of the disease. First of all, the family should contact the Alzheimer's Association (AA), which can offer needed management advice through personal contact, literature, and videos. The AA will typically recommend establishing and following a strict daily schedule, which the SLP can help the family get started. Through extensive use of calendars, clocks, pictures, and notepads, the family and patient can develop ways of following a routine schedule. The SLP will encourage the patient to attend a support group, meeting with other memory loss patients in social situations. Old movies and video shows are often appreciated, as well as listening to and singing old musical favorites. Photographs and videos of favorite vacation spots often stimulate conversation, particularly among those people who actually had been there. A skillful group leader can weave past situations into fun participation by most members of a dementia group. While the people with dementia are socializing in their group, family members often meet in a family-support group. Family group meetings offer family members the psychological support they need for coping with the drastic changes they are experiencing with their loved one's increasing dementia.

The SLP also can offer activities the patient can do at home. Nonverbal activities like solving Sudoku puzzles or completing pictorial jigsaw puzzles can expand the patient's attention span. The SLP can set up particular verbal and nonverbal computer apps that the patient can do with only minimal family assistance. In general, verbal analogies and fragmented discourse should be avoided. The dementia patient often enjoys working alone without spoken instructions. The Alzheimer's Association recognizes patient success in attending to nonverbal tasks and has collected a number of performance tasks the SLP can set up for families to use at home.

Cerebral Palsy

Although two people with cerebral palsy, Ed and Bonnie, have tales in this book, cerebral palsy is not a typical disorder treated by an SLP in a medical setting. Rather, I included them in *Trouble Talking* because each of their stories has an important lesson for any us meeting or working with severely motor-handicapped people. Ed, for example, with his flailing athetoid movements appeared that he would have major problems speaking. He did not. He surprised us all with his clear thinking and well-articulated sentences. His story offers a warning: Don't prejudge one's intellect or verbal ability only by their appearance or diagnostic label.

Bonnie, a teenager with a severe spastic athetoid motor problem, died unexpectedly during a surgical procedure. I had worked closely with Bonnie as her SLP for many months, but also spent time sharing pictures of my wife and baby and interacting socially with Bonnie and her mother. Her death was a shock to me. It did teach me an important lesson: When we perform in our professional roles with a patient, it's advisable to avoid getting too emotionally involved with that person.

The term *cerebral palsy* (CP) comes from the brain's *cerebrum*, which regulates motor function, and the word *palsy*, which labels the paralysis of voluntary movement. According to the Cerebral Palsy Foundation, cerebral palsy occurs when there is neurological damage before, during, or within five years after birth.

Treatment of motor feeding problems, if present, begins early in infancy. The overall treatment of sensory-motor problems in the infant and young child with cerebral palsy may begin in the hospital but soon transfers to outpatient CP clinics. With heavy focus on preschool development, the child and family work closely with members of the CP rehabilitation teams: child development specialists, physical and occupational therapists, and the SLP. In the school-age years, there will ideally be a well-staffed special education program that will help the child continue to develop greater motor control and achieve future academic success.

Apraxia

In apraxia, the patient cannot perform a motor task when asked to do so. For example, with arm apraxia, when we ask a patient to catch a ball, he cannot move his hands to make the catch. If we suddenly throw a ball without announcing it, he'll reach out and catch it immediately. Apraxia is the inability to perform a motor task on purpose contrasted with the normal ability to do so automatically. Rose, our Parkinson's patient, suffered from gait apraxia. When asked to make a step forward, she could not move her leg to do so. Only when we found a way of coupling the command with automatic walking was she able to step forward into an elevator. Frank displayed an odd form of ideomotor apraxia illustrated by an inability to sit down upon request, contrasted by normal automatic sitting when not requested to sit. If someone said or made a hand gesture to sit, Frank was immediately aware of his inability to sit on command, and he would say something like, "I wish you hadn't said that."

The apraxia shown by both Rose and Frank eventually disappeared without therapy. Oral apraxias are rare but can be treated effectively by the SLP using methods developed in treating expressive aphasia patients.[5] There is little literature available on the treatment of other forms of apraxia. Fortunately, the patient can still perform automatic arm and leg movements during the time he waits for the usually spontaneous reduction of the apraxia and return to normal motor function.

Head Trauma

It is difficult to generalize about head trauma. As discussed in chapter 1, while we could locate different kinds of aphasia by CVA or trauma to particular sections of the left cerebral hemisphere, symptoms of brain injury are as diverse as the type, location, and severity of the trauma. Only three of the tales in this book were about people with head trauma: Louie with a left hemisphere bullet wound, Captain Bill with right hemisphere trauma, and Josh. Our 22-year-old Josh apparently experienced right-sided head trauma, which left him with a few language confusions and a slight left arm paresis.

For Josh and other new head trauma patients, soon after the head trauma occurs, the patient and family will have their first contact with an SLP, who will examine for any communication disorders, such as hearing loss, language deficits, and dysarthria. Dysarthria is a motor speech disorder experienced by many of our people in the neurogenic tales. Dysarthria can show itself in many different ways: slurred articulation, changes in speaking rate, and voice resonance changes. The treatment of dysarthria by the SLP is then started if any speech deficits are found. The head trauma patient will be evaluated by several medical specialists, such as neurologists, neuropsychiatrists, and physiatrists. Josh met several times with the hospital neuropsychologist, who was most helpful to both Josh and his mother in managing a few of his perceptual concerns.

Parkinson's Disease

According to the Parkinson's Disease Foundation (PDF), nearly one million people in the United State are living with Parkinson's disease (PD). The first symptom is often a non-intention tremor of one or both hands. When the hand is at rest there is tremor, but when intentionally reaching for something the tremor disappears. This was our PD patient Phyllis's first symptom. Her non-intention tremor at rest would stop with any kind of intentional motor movement. As PD symptoms progress, there is an increase in slowness of movements, such as small shuffling steps when walking. Handwriting becomes smaller. Of some concern is a growing impairment of balance and coordination, often requiring a cane for safe ambulation. Soft-spoken and slurred speech develops, with patients reporting that they "are often asked to repeat what they just said."

Human speech and voice when we talk are automatic motor behaviors.[6] We don't know if our soft palate is open or shut, or if our vocal folds are together, or how our tongue is moving within our mouth, and so forth. Like other automatic motor behaviors, speech production comes fast without any deliberation. Much of automatic motor function is controlled and executed by large bilateral structures in the lower part of the brain, known as the *basal ganglia*. Some nerve tracts from the cortex pass by the basal ganglia without stopping, which permits deliberate and intentional motor acts. For example, the game of basketball illustrates a comparison of automatic versus deliberate motor tasks: Dribbling down the court dodging defenders is a highly automatic behavior; in contrast, shooting a basket from the free-throw line is a study of deliberation.

The passage of nerve impulses to, within, and from the basal ganglia is facilitated by a substance known as *dopamine*. This micro-fluid is vital for the normal transmission of nerve impulses required for normal motor movements Lack of sufficient dopamine is the primary cause of the symptoms of Parkinson's disease. Laboratory testing of many PD patients often reveals drastic reductions from normal dopamine levels. Medications that facilitate greater dopamine production are the drug treatments of choice in PD.

Behavioral deficits in Parkinson's are best treated by therapy. The SLP plays a vital role in improving the speech and voice of the Parkinson's patient. In the 1950s, in a chronic disease rehabilitation hospital, a dramatic contrast in speech intelligibility was noted between when PD patients were asked to count forward, from 1 to 15, and then backward, from 15 to 1. The automatic motor task of forward counting often resulted in soft loudness and mumbled speech. Apparently, reverse counting used greater intention, shown by louder, more articulate speech. The muscles used for breathing and oral motor function receive a "better workout" when speaking with greater intention. Translating these findings to increasing intent with therapy, we practiced these techniques: slowing down speaking rate, speaking with a pretend accent, speaking louder, and exaggerating the pronunciation of the last syllable of a word. Our PD patient Rose practiced all four of these techniques in therapy. Years later, we found that speaking much louder was the easiest of the techniques to do. Therefore, in our speaking-with-intent therapy with Phyllis, priority was given to her producing a louder voice and using intent by measuring her loudness levels.

The patient and family search for a certified SLP might be started by contacting the Michael J. Fox Foundation, which is always searching for improved PD therapies. Also, the ASHA ProFind program can take a patient's name and provide the names of SLPs and possible speech clinic possibilities in the patient's home community.

There are several national and international Parkinson's rehabilitation programs for improving speech and voice that use louder voice as their primary focus in therapy. Loudness is measured in therapy with sound level meters to help the patient maintain his or her focus on intent, not allowing the practice task to be produced as a wholly automatic motor response. The usual goal of speech therapy for most disorders is to encourage carryover to automatic production. Not in speech therapy for Parkinson's. Parkinson's therapy is effective when *never* creating automatic carryover, but always using deliberate motor movements as a method for keeping therapy intention. Louder voice seems to encourage more vigorous muscle participation, which in turn prevents muscle atrophy and encourages muscle strength. For the PD patient, a spinoff from increasing muscle strength and function while swallowing is that aspiration of fluids and food is mostly eliminated.

Most SLPs are trained to use specific PD therapy programs. The patient is often scheduled for individual therapy for three to four sessions weekly. The number of total required therapy sessions varies with the program. One program requires 16 individual sessions over a four- to five-week period, followed by once-weekly group meetings. Another major program requires continuous therapy until the patient meets an established dismissal criteria; the patient starts group therapy in the beginning of individual therapy and after discharge from individual therapy, and continues in a group for as long as he or she wishes. Phyllis, for example, has continued in her Parkinson's therapy group for over five years.

Friedreich's Ataxia

The symptoms of Friedreich's ataxia (FA) do not show in childhood until between 5 to 15 years of age. As an inherited disease, the spinal cord and peripheral nerves degenerate causing a host of sensory-motor problems. Alice in our "Robin Hood" tale showed the first symptoms at age nine, with severe gait ataxia emerging including imbalance trying to walk. She later experienced severe involvement of facial and neck muscles and lost most functional ability to use her arms and hands. Breathing difficulties and deterioration of facial muscle function gradually contributed to deterioration of her speech. Although now at age 44, she continued to try to improve her speech; "inside her head" she appeared to have normal language.

As with many degenerative diseases of the nervous system, there is currently no cure for FA. However, as a welcomed speech patient in a university speech clinic, Alice could show functional speech and feeding improvement from time to time. As symptoms temporarily lessened, Alice would work closely with her university student clinician and make some temporary gains.

Amyotrophic Lateral Sclerosis

At 51 years of age, our tennis pro, Mike, began to experience the first symptoms of amyotrophic lateral sclerosis (ALS), popularly known as Lou Gehrig's disease. Gehrig was a Yankee baseball hero who in his mid-30s began to experience some numbness and weakness running to first base, the beginning symptoms of his progressive neurological disease (ALS). Gehrig was a few years younger than the typical age of onset of ALS, which is usually between ages 40 and 60. Typical of leg weakness being an early symptom of ALS, Mike's increasing leg weakness forced him off the tennis courts. Anyone who begins to experience the early symptoms of leg weakness should immediately see their personal physician, who will make appropriate referrals to a neurologist. If ALS is the diagnosis, the patient or family can contact the Amyotrophic Lateral Sclerosis Association (ALSA) for help and long-term guidance. Founded in 1985, the ALS Association offers families needed literature and counseling about the disorder and personal help in finding appropriate therapy.

According to the ALSA, the typical projected lifespan after the onset of ALS symptoms is only two to four years. The leg muscles start with some stiffness, followed by muscle atrophy with a noticeable decrease in muscle size. The disease progresses with atrophy of bilateral arm and hand muscles, eventually involving oral muscles, seriously affecting the muscles of mastication and swallowing. Oral muscle involvement presents a continuing challenge to the SLP. In the beginning of Mike's facial and tongue involvement, he was able to extend the clarity of his speech by intensive reading aloud of word-lists designed to focus on particular muscle movements. In his final weeks of life, Mike experienced an increasing pooling of mucus and liquid in the bottom of his throat. Throat clearing was supplemented by his wife and nurses, using syringes to suction fluids out when needed. Like most other ALS patients, Mike's death (three years after onset) came from fluid aspiration.

Voice Disorders

If anyone experiences a sudden change of voice that lasts for more than a week, that person should have a medical examination of the mouth, throat, and larynx, hopefully by an ear, nose, and throat (ENT) physician (otolaryngologist). After our review of a number of diseases that might affect voice and speech, one can appreciate why early identification and appropriate medical management is needed. Faulty changes in voice (dysphonia) are often found to be produced by a normal larynx and vocal folds, which categorizes the voice disorder as a *functional dysphonia*. The ENT refers such a patient to the SLP for voice evaluation and possible voice therapy.

A large number of voice problems come from both children and adults misusing their voices. In chapter 4, "Tales of Voice Disorders," we looked at several people who had been misusing their voices. The story about Tom, the lawyer, demonstrated the chewing technique used with patients who do not open their mouths enough as they speak, one technique the SLP uses as treatment for functional dysphonia. Penny's continuous yelling and occasional screaming eventually produced bilateral vocal nodules that produced a hoarse voice. Once the nodules were removed surgically, Penny began successful voice therapy, which led to replacing her functional dysphonia to an "easy-to-listen-to voice." The basketball coach Fred was extreme in his use of vocal hyperfunction, losing his voice completely after a basketball game. Fortunately, he was successful in voice therapy, reducing his yelling and eliminating his hoarse voice. The coach found that if he must yell, he had to learn how to do it.

Some voice patients self-refer themselves to the SLP over concern they may have about their voices. Catherine, a book editor in a major publishing house, was concerned that her high, baby-sounding voice did not match her needs for a more confident-sounding authoritarian voice. Through voice therapy, she was able to develop and use a deeper, more resonant voice, a voice that clearly met her professional needs. Over the years of telephone follow-up, Catherine liked to "scare" her old SLP by intentionally speaking a few words with her old voice. Then she would revert back to her now well-established professional voice.

Thornton, concerned about his high voice after his excessive-chlorine accident, was thankful that voice therapy helped to reduce his high voice pitch to slightly lower levels. Other voice patients may show some concern about their functional voice problems, but their concern is never matched by any self-practice using suggested voice remediation techniques. Wanda was such a patient. Her voice concerns were no match to replace her overwhelming concern for the plight of the birds in Denver.

Carl in the state prison fainted after a traumatic event, awakened, and was unable to find his voice or speech. His loss of voice was not a voice problem per se, but a form of conversion aphonia (APA 2013). Despite having normal speech and voice mechanisms, the patient's reaction to a specific traumatic event was the inability to "find" his voice. With counseling and strong psychological support, such patients usually recover their normal voices.

Our two laryngectomy patients, Harvey and Roberta, both had laryngeal cancer, requiring a total laryngectomy. Their voice surgical procedures were quite different, requiring distinctively different training procedures for acquiring an esophageal voice. Harvey's operation over 50 years ago separated his airway from his esophagus. He breathed through an opening in his neck called a tracheotomy. His new voice came from swallowing and trapping air in his esophagus and bringing it up as a continuous belch for his substitute voice. Roberta benefited from more recent surgical procedures that connected her airway through a vent directly to the esophagus. By placing her finger directly over the tracheotomy, her outgoing air stream was sent directly to her esophagus, providing all the air she needed for producing a good esophageal voice.

Both Harvey and Roberta developed excellent esophageal voices. Also, having good outgoing personalities, they made excellent models for new laryngectomy patients to visit with shortly before and after their surgeries.

Stuttering

Most of the patient tales in *Trouble Talking* are stories about people seen by the SLP in medical settings. The three tales of Ronnie, Eric, and Dr. John came from situations monitored in university speech clinics. Ronnie was only five years old when he was first evaluated with a stuttering problem so severe that he had no functional speech. His positive reaction to a unique beginning of treatment was why this five-year-old's story, "Pith Helmet Therapy," was included in this volume.

Ronnie by age five had experienced several years trying to speak against his severe problem of stuttering. There was no melody-flow, or prosody, to anything he attempted to say. An oral examination and observations of him chewing foods and swallowing solids and liquids revealed normal mechanisms capable of producing normal speech. After asking him to repeat different-sounding jargon sounds, his SLP was surprised at how quickly Ronnie was able to do this.

Pith helmet therapy, or using "jungle words," came about from his normal ability to produce nonsense sounds, using his mouth to speak without experiencing struggle. After several jargon therapy sessions, Ronnie was able to produce some normal forward speech, enabling him to bridge into more traditional therapy. Ronnie and his family followed many of the therapy methods and controls offered by the Stuttering Foundation of America (SFA, 2017). Founded in 1947, with the logo "Helping Those Who Stutter," Ronnie has been an active supporter of the SFA for over 40 years.

Eric, our ship captain, has had a lifetime of speech therapy for his stuttering. Eric said in group therapy that the day as a teenager he learned to stop avoiding his stuttering was the day he no longer feared stuttering. He stopped fearing certain words and finding substitutes for those words he knew he could not say. Instead, he would plunge ahead and use a few methods he had learned for saying any feared word. In going forward with speaking, Eric used his positive thinking the same way as when he goes forward with confidence in "parking" a ship.

Dr. John was an established SLP who had experienced a lifetime as someone who stuttered. Over the years, he had profited from speech therapy. After years of therapy and graduate school education, his speech was good enough that he headed the speech clinic of a major university, taught undergraduate and graduate courses, provided clinical supervision, and conducted speech-related research. When I first met Dr. John, he had only one flaw in his overall performance—he stuttered badly on the land phone. However, when visiting him, I observed him to be reasonably fluent on his cell phone. He had learned to stutter on the only phone available for most of his life, the land phone. After my visit, by using an operant approach, he had desensitized his reactions to a conventional phone. Dr. John recently called me and went out of his way to let me know he was speaking on a land phone. His speech was normal.

A Final Comment

Communication disorders are many and varied—as are the people who have them. They may have problems that interfere with their understanding of what others say, or less visible problems in not understanding what they read. Their difficulties using normal language, speech, and voice may cause a serious compromise in communication between speaker and listener. Our portrayals of communication disorders have shown this compromise in our brief tales, some humorous and some sad. Over the years, successful treatment of communication disorders has grown markedly through the efforts of rehabilitation specialists including the speech-language pathologist, medical specialists, special educators, the family, and, just as importantly, by the people with the problem.

~

Notes

Introduction

1. Thomas Wolfe, *The Kingdom of Speech* (New York: Little, Brown & Company, 2016).

2. Oliver Sacks, *The Man Who Mistook His Wife for a Hat* (New York: Touchstone, 1998).

Chapter 5: Tales of Speech Pathology

1. Thomas Wolfe, *The Kingdom of Speech* (New York: Little, Brown & Company, 2016)

Chapter 6: Management of Communication Disorders

1. Richard C. Senelick, *Living with Stroke*, 4th ed. (New York: McGraw-Hill, 2010).

2. Dalia Cahana-Amitay and Martin Albert, *Redefining Recovery from Aphasia* (Oxford University Press, 2015).

3. Kathryn Bayles and Daniel R. Boone, *Journal of Speech and Hearing Research* (1982), 10–217.

4. Elena M. Plante and Pelagie M. Beeson, *Communication and Communication Disorders*, 4th ed. (Boston: Pearson Education, 2012).

5. Leonard L. LaPointe, *Paul Broca and the Origins of Language in the Brain* (San Diego: Plural Publishing, 2013).

6. Daniel R. Boone, et al., *The Voice and Voice Therapy*, 9th ed. (Boston: Pearson Education, 2013).

~

Bibliography

APA, *Diagnostic and Statistical Manual of Mental Disorders*, 5th ed. (Washington, DC: American Psychiatric Association, 2013).

Bayles, Kathryn A., and Daniel R. Boone, "The Potential of Language Tasks for Identifying Senile Dementia, *Journal of Speech and Hearing Disorders*, 47: 210–217 (1982).

Boone, Daniel R., *Is Your Voice Telling on You?* 3rd ed. (San Diego: Plural Publishing, 2016).

Boone, Daniel R., et al., *The Voice and Voice Therapy*, 9th ed. (Boston: Pearson Education, 2013).

Byrd, Courtney T., *What I Wish People Knew About Stuttering* (The Stuttering Foundation, 2010).

Cahana-Amitay, Dalia, and Martin Albert, *Redefining Recovery from Aphasia* (New York: Oxford University Press, 2015).

LaPointe, Leonard L., *Paul Broca and the Origins of Language in the Brain* (San Diego: Plural Publishing, 2013).

Plante, Elena M., and Pelagie M. Beeson, *Communication and Communication Disorders*, 4th ed. (Boston: Pearson Education, 2012).

Sacks, Oliver, *The Man Who Mistook His Wife for a Hat* (New York: Touchstone, 1998).

Schum, Richard L., *Clinical Perspectives on the Treatment of Selective Mutism* (APA PsycNET, Vol. 1, No. 2, Summer 2006).

Senelick, Richard C., *Living with Stroke*, 4th ed. (New York: McGraw-Hill, 2010).

Wolfe, Thomas, *The Kingdom of Speech* (New York: Little, Brown & Company, 2016).

~

Resources

Readers can contact these family-friendly organizations for further information about the communication problems discussed in this book.

Alzheimer's Association
225 North Michigan Avenue, Floor 17
Chicago, IL 60601
(800) 272-3900
www.alz.org
The AA was founded in 1980 and offers resources in Alzheimer's care, support, and research.

American Speech-Language-Hearing Association
2200 Research Boulevard
Rockville, MD 20850
(800) 638-8255
www.asha.org
ASHA was founded in 1925 and is the national professional, scientific, and credentialing association for audiologists, speech-language pathologists, and speech scientists. Its mission is making effective communication accessible and achievable for all.

Amyotrophic Lateral Sclerosis Association
1275 K Street NW, Suite 250
Washington, DC 20005
(202) 407-8580
www.alsa.org

The ALS Association was founded in 1985 to raise money for research and patient services, promote awareness about, and advocate in state and federal government on issues related to ALS.

Brain Injury Association of America
1608 Spring Hill Road, Suite 110
Vienna, VA 22182
(800) 444-6443
www.biausa.org

BIAA's mission, since 1980, is to advance awareness, research, and treatment for those who have experienced traumatic brain injury.

Cerebral Palsy Foundation
3 Columbus Circle, 15th Floor
New York, NY 10019
(212) 520-1686
www.yourcpf.org

The CPF was founded in 1948 to serve individuals and their families with cerebral palsy by bringing together experts in medicine, counseling, and technology.

Mental Health America
(800) 273-8255
www.mentalhealthamerica.net

The MHA was founded in 1909 and is the nation's leading community-based nonprofit dedicated to those living with mental illness and vascular dementia.

Michael J. Fox Foundation
469 7th Avenue, Suite 498
New York, NY 10018
(800) 708-7644
www.michaeljfox.org

The Michael J. Fox Foundation for Parkinson's Research was founded in 2000 and is dedicated to finding a cure for Parkinson's disease through funded research and ensuring the development of improved therapies for those living with Parkinson's today.

Multiple Dystrophy Association
222 South Riverside Plaza, Suite 1500
Chicago, IL 60606
(800) 572-1717
www.mda.org
   The MDA was founded in 1950 and is committed to curing multiple dystrophy, ALS, and related diseases by funding worldwide research.

National Aphasia Association
350 7th Avenue, Suite 902
New York, NY 10001
(212) 267-2814
www.aphasia.org
   The NAA was founded in 1987 and advocates for persons with aphasia and their families.

National Association of Teachers of Singing
9957 Moorings Drive #401
Jacksonville, FL 32257
(904) 992-9101
www.info@nats.org
   NATS was founded in 1944 and is the largest professional association of teachers of singing in the world.

National Multiple Sclerosis Society
1700 Owens Street
San Francisco, CA 94158
(800) 344-4867
www.nationalmssociety.org
   The NMSS was founded in 1946 and supports and connects people with multiple sclerosis with health care providers, volunteers, donors, and others who seek a world free of MS.

Parkinson's Disease Foundation
1359 Broadway, Suite 1509
New York, NY 10018
(212) 923-4700
www.pdf.org
   The PDF was founded in 1957 to find a cure for Parkinson's disease and ensure the best quality of life for those who live with the disease.

The Stuttering Foundation of America
P.O. Box 11749
Memphis, TN 38111-0749
(800) 992-9392 or (901) 761-0343
www.stutteringhelp.org

The SFA was founded in 1947 and provides support and information to the stuttering community.

Voice and Speech Trainers Association
(773) 888-2782
www.vasta.org

Founded in 1950, VASTA is dedicated to serving the needs of the voice and speech profession and to developing the art and science of the human voice.

webMD
1201 Peachtree Street NE
Atlanta, GA 30301
www.customercare.webmd.com

Founded in 1996, webMD is a leading source of timely health and medical news and information (hard copy, email, and online).

~

About the Author

Daniel R. Boone, PhD, is a professor emeritus in the Department of Speech, Language, and Hearing Sciences at the University of Arizona. He has published seventeen books and more than one hundred other publications (chapters and articles) on voice and aphasia, motor speech, and voice disorders. He is revered nationally and internationally for his teaching and clinical activities as well as for his love and dedication to his students, and he is a household name to all who study speech pathology.

Dr. Boone, who belongs to the "group of founding fathers of American speech pathology," is sought after as a speaker, lecturer, and workshop leader on voice disorders, communication problems in aging, and new perspectives in speech pathology. He is a former president of the American Speech-Language-Hearing Association and a recipient of both Fellowship and Honors from that organization, as well as many other honors and recognitions. He serves on numerous editorial boards of scholarly journals and contributes regularly to research literature. Dr. Boone continues to offer voice therapy workshops for the Parkinson Voice Project in Dallas, Texas, and serves as a voice and motor speech consultant at his studio in Tucson, Arizona.